management essentials in nursing

claire b. keane, b.s., r.n., m.ed.

reston publishing company, inc.
a prentice-hall company
reston, virginia

Library of Congress Cataloging in Publication Data

Keane, Claire Brackman,
    Management Essentials in Nursing.

    Includes bibliographies and index.
    1.   Nursing service administration.   I.   Title.
[DNLM: 1.   Nursing, Supervisory—Organization and
administration. WY105 K24m]
RT89.K42   610.73'068   80-22654
ISBN 0-8359-4203-1
ISBN 0-8359-4202-3 (pbk.)

preface

Management is a glorious mixture of intangible qualities and tangible quantities. As a concept it exists only in the minds of people; as a reality it is evidenced in every aspect of our lives. Theories related to the practice of management come from every discipline; guidelines for applying these theories most often come from the men and women who apply the theories in the real world of work. Practicing managers, like professional practitioners in every profession, must depend on a combination of intellect and intuition to accomplish the goals that are important to them and to the society in which they live and work.

The purpose of this book is to present some of the theoretical and pragmatic bases for the practice of management in a health-care setting. A health-care organization is viewed here as a highly complex system that attempts to maintain equilibrium in a dynamic and changing environment. The notions of system, process, structure, and equilibrium should not be new to a nurse-manager. We will attempt to point out how many of these concepts that are basic to the practice of nursing are applicable also to the practice of management.

The management of a system as complex as the human body requires an ability to see the person as a whole composed of physiologic, psychologic, and sociologic subsystems that are in a continual state of flux. One cannot deal effectively with one aspect of an integrated living system that is a human being without considering each of the other aspects of the person's life. The manager of a patient care unit faces a similar situation when he/she engages in the management process. The organization must be seen as a viable system that cannot survive without integration and coordination of all the activities that take place in the various departments that are the subsystems of the organization. The activities of a first-line manager have impact on all the variables of the system and its subsystems. These variables include the individuals working in the patient care unit and throughout the organization, the interpersonal interactions among these individuals, and the interaction of human behavior, attitudes, and values, with the bureaucratic structure and missions, goals, and purposes of the organization.

It is difficult to isolate each of these variables and reorganize information about them into a logical sequence. The manner in which this has been done in this text will not meet the approval of every reader and there will be no attempt on the part of the author to defend the organization and sequencing. We begin with an overview of the historical development of management thought and the contributions of various disciplines to the formation of organizational theory. We then turn our attention to the process of management and to the activities performed within the roles of the nurse-manager.

The activities of decision making, motivating, leading, and communicating pervade every aspect of the management process. These are treated separately in Chapters 4 through 7, but in reality they cannot be divided. They are so closely interrelated and interdependent it is impossible for the practicing manager to attend to one without having some impact on each of the others.

The evaluation of employee performance also is a pervasive influence in the management of people. Chapter 10 attempts to show how a participative and humanistic appraisal of subordinates can help develop the potential of every employee and improve the quality of care provided to patients and clients.

Limitations of space prohibit an individual acknowledgement to each of the persons who have contributed to this manuscript. Without their continued support, suggestions, advice, and encouragement this book could not exist. Having been singularly blessed with good friends and competent helpers, I thank their God and mine for the gifts of their time and talents.

Claire B. Keane
Athens, Georgia

contents

chapter 1
index

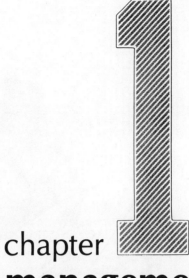

chapter

what is management?

Management is an abstract word, an idea, an intangible that exists only in the minds of people. Because it is intangible and highly complex, most of us define management in terms of outcome. For example, we say that an orderly household, a successful business, or a winning football team is well managed. Sometimes in their desperation to define an abstract term such as management, people will resort to the cliche, "I can't tell you exactly what it is, but I know it when I see it."

Most textbook definitions of management include at least three factors that help determine the outcome of the management process: (1) the objectives, (2) the people involved, and (3) the organization. Successful managers of any kind of enterprise requiring the cooperative effort of people do not do the work themselves; they get it done through other people under their guidance and direction.

In the process of managing, the manager deals with three elements: *things, people,* and *ideas*. In his classic three-dimensional model of the management process, MacKenzie places these three elements at the core of the process, with all of the management tasks, functions and activities orbiting around them.[1] (See Figure 1.1.)

If you were to rate each of the three elements according to the ease with which they can be handled, you probably would rate *things* as the least difficult and *ideas* as the most difficult elements. Ideas or concepts are intangibles that have a way of slipping by us, going over our heads as it were, because we have difficulty sending and receiving messages about what they mean. It is essential that you know at least some of the terminology commonly used in writings that explain or describe the many aspects of management.

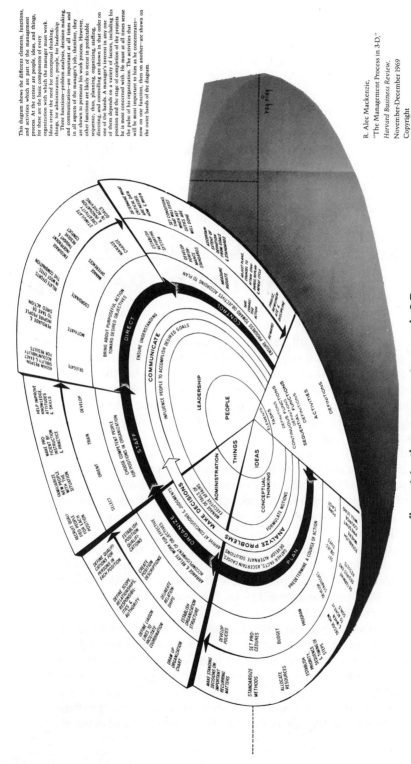

This diagram shows the different elements, functions, and activities which are part of the management process. At the center are people, ideas, and things, for these are the basic components of every organization with which the manager must work. Ideas create the need for conceptual thinking, things, for administration; people, for leadership.

Three functions—problem analysis, decision making, and communication—are important at all times and in all aspects of the manager's job; therefore, they are shown to permeate his work process. However, other functions are likely to occur in predictable sequence; thus, planning, organizing, staffing, directing, and controlling are shown in that order on one of the bands. A manager's interest in any one of them depends on a variety of factors, including his position and the stage of completion of the projects he is most concerned with. He must at all times sense the pulse of his organization. The activities that will be most important to him as he concentrates—now on one function, then on another—are shown on the outer bands of the diagram.

R. Alec Mackenzie,
"The Management Process in 3-D,"
Harvard Business Review,
November–December 1969
Copyright

figure 1.1   the management process in 3-D

In this chapter we will attempt to clarify some of the key concepts in management, tracing their development through the years. We will also identify some of the leaders in the field and tell how they have influenced even to the present organization theory and the practice of management.

From the earliest studies of management and the things people do when they manage, there has been a general consensus about the basic functions of management. In the first half of the twentieth century Henri Fayol, a French industrialist, proposed a general theory of management that he believed to be applicable in any organizational setting. Fayol identified five basic functions of management: *planning, organizing, commanding, coordinating,* and *controlling.*[2] Refinements and revisions of this list of functions are found throughout management literature.

The three-dimensional model developed by MacKenzie in the 1960's shows five management functions that are not too different from Fayol's list. MacKenzie sees these functions as being more or less sequential. The process begins when the manager identifies some goals and objectives and starts *planning* for their achievement. The next function is *organizing* the work into manageable units, and then *staffing* or selecting people to do the work. The manager then *directs* or guides the activities of staff members, and finally, uses such methods of *control* as evaluation of the outcome of the process and appraisal of staff performance to determine whether the goals and objectives have been met.[3]

Throughout the remainder of this text we will explore more fully your tasks and responsibilities in performance of the sequential functions of management and the ongoing activities of communicating, problem solving, and decision making in the management process. (See Figure 1.2.)

ORGANIZATION THEORY AND MANAGEMENT SCIENCE

Organization theory is that body of knowledge that serves as a foundation for the practice of management. It is a large and diverse collection of information obtained through the efforts of researchers and scientists in such disciplines as economics, sociology, anthropology, psychology, political science, and philosophy.

While these contributions have greatly enriched and expanded the field of management, they also have added to its complexity, making it difficult to present the topic of management as an integrated and unified whole. Ironically, although management itself is concerned with integration and orderly progress toward objectives, it almost defies attempts to organize and integrate its own subject matter.

There continues to be some controversy over whether or not management is a science and a profession and whether it does indeed have a body of knowledge that is entirely its own. We will leave that to the experts. For our

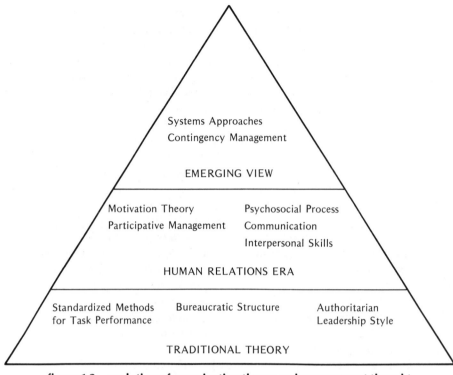

figure 1.2   evolution of organization theory and management thought

purposes we will use the phrase *management science* for convenience rather than as an indication that it qualifies as a recognized science among more fully researched and developed fields of study.

Some of the earliest writings on management came from men who recorded their observations and experiences as executives and administrators in industry. The contribution of practicing managers who have first hand experience with the problems of management continues to be a source of information for students and practitioners. In the latter part of the nineteenth century, engineers and economists began to conduct time and motion studies and analyses of tasks performed by workers, and devise methods of operation that would increase productivity and decrease time and effort. Their recommendations for improving efficiency in industrial operations were the beginning of traditional or classical organization theory.

TRADITIONAL CONCEPTS OF MANAGEMENT

If we were to divide the development of management thought into three phases (see Figure 1.2), the first phase would begin at about the time of the industrial revolution and the formation of large scale industrial organizations such as those in the automobile and railroad industries. During this phase the scientific principles of management were first formulated and the so-called *scientific management* school of thought developed.

During this era executives of organizations were chiefly concerned with *things*. Pioneers such as Frederick W. Taylor, considered the father of scientific management, believed that the function of management was to provide specific guidelines for the performance of work. They would *enforce* standardized methods, *enforce* adoption of the most efficient means of accomplishing a task, and *enforce* cooperation from the workers so that the work could be done more quickly.[4]

Some of the assumptions made by traditional theorists about the nature of man and his attitudes toward work are reflected in their suggestions for improvement in the practice of management. Among these assumptions were the beliefs that there is "one best way" to perform every task, that workers require close supervision and detailed instructions and strict controls to ensure their cooperation in meeting organizational goals, and that a formal hierarchy is needed for the coordination of tasks.[5]

In this period of history an authoritarian style of management was thought to be the only effective way to get the job done. The needs of employees, if they were considered at all, were certainly secondary to the goals of the organization. It was assumed that people work for money and that salary was the most important motivator to get them to work harder toward organizational goals.

As a first-line manager, you benefit from the work of traditional theorists of management. Without them there would be no policies or standardized procedures for evaluating work performance, no departmental divisions of work, and none of the structural characteristics of organizations that we take for granted today. Although traditional concepts of management are chiefly authoritarian and highly structured, they continue to be valid alternatives in certain kinds of management situations.

Some of the concepts that developed from the traditional era probably are familiar to you, though some may not be. We will discuss these now so that you might have a better understanding of what is meant by *task performance, efficiency and effectiveness, bureaucratic structure,* and *structure and process* in a management situation.

task performance

The word *task*, according to *Webster's Third International Dictionary* refers to "a specific piece of work or service, usually imposed by authority or circumstances." In its broader sense, a task is a duty, responsibility, or assignment. In management literature the author may intend to convey either the more specific definition or the broader usage, depending on the context in which it is written.

The organization of work and division of labor may be oriented toward a *whole-task* or a *part-task* system of assignment. For example, nursing is a task in the more general sense; it is a duty, and responsibility accepted by members of the profession. The *primary nursing* system of assignments is more of a whole-task approach than is the assignment of nursing care teams who divide the work into more specific tasks or procedures. Some members of the nursing team might give all of the medications, for example, while others share other responsibilities of nursing care.

In general, professional health care personnel are better satisfied with a whole-task system of work organization than are technical workers. However, all levels of workers need to feel they have made a significant contribution toward achieving the goals and objectives of nursing care. The more divisions made in the whole task of nursing, the more difficult it is for employees to see how they have influenced the quality of the service provided through their efforts. There are some who would argue that this kind of fragmentation is in the long run less effective and less conducive to accountability, acceptance of responsibility, and the professional growth of individuals.

Kramer suggests that one of the causes of disenchantment among new graduates of schools of professional nursing is the conflict that arises from their expectations about performing whole-task nursing as they were taught in school, and the expectations of nurse-employing organizations. Traditionally, these organizations have shown a preference for a part-task system for the division of work.[6]

efficiency and effectiveness

Early management scientists such as Taylor and his followers concentrated their studies on improving the speed with which a task could be done with the least possible expenditure of human and material resources. Although they were successful to some degree, the incentive wages given for faster production were not as effective as they might have hoped. Changing operations so that work is done more efficiently is helpful, but eventually one reaches a point of maximum benefit from speed and organized performance of a job.

We do not measure efficiency and effectiveness by exactly the same criteria, even though they are equally important in accomplishing the goals of an organization in which cost is a factor. The rising costs of health care remind us that managers at every level must be attentive to the efficient use of resources and prevention of waste. However, these concerns should be balanced with attention to the short-term and long-term effects of the services and products so efficiently produced. Probably the criteria of efficiency will be met by the punctual performance of nursing procedures, a minimal expenditure of energy and money, and compliance with rules, policies, and standard procedures of the hospital or clinic. On the other hand, it is possible that the procedures may not be as effective as they could be, insofar as the patients or clients are concerned. The art of nursing and the art of management require something more than cold and dispassionate efficiency. While efficiency is always desirable in nursing care, effectiveness is critical to successful outcome.

bureaucratic structure

An important contribution to classical or traditional organization theory was the bureaucratic model developed by Max Weber, a German sociologist whose writings were influential during the early 1920's. In recent years the word *bureaucracy* has fallen on hard times, but in Weber's day it was accepted with enthusiasm, chiefly because it provided a more rational and less whimsical basis for many administrative decisions and for establishing lines of authority. The notion of authority by virtue of position on the hierarchical scale came from the model of bureaucracy, just as the promotion and selection of personnel, especially managers, was based on aptitude for the job.

Critics of the bureaucratic model point out that so much regimentation stifles creativity and deprives employees of opportunities to be innovative and effective in bringing about needed change. Although rules, standards and other evidence of formal structure are necessary, it is suggested that the bureaucratic model is most appropriate when routine activities must be carried out.

structure and process

It was also in the 1920's that Mary Parker Follett conceptualized the organization as a *social system* in which the people doing the work were as worthy of the attention of the manager as were the "things." She defined the essence of management as "getting things done through people" and thus established a link between the mechanistic traditional era and the human relations period of management history.[7]

If one considers the organization as a *social system* and the exercise of management as a *social process,* then the manager's concerns must extend beyond formal structure to interpersonal relationships, communication, leadership, and other less tangible and more dynamic variables in the process. Comparing and contrasting formal structure and process is not the same as viewing them as opposing aspects of a system. They are both essential and relevant to the accomplishment of objectives.

In general, formal structure refers to the arrangement of the components of a system and their relationship to one another. They are roughly analogous to the anatomical components of a biologic system in the body. Structure is usually thought of as being static, relatively stable, and slow to respond to forces for change. Examples of formal structure in an organization might include organizational charts showing lines of authority or chain of command and areas of responsibility, job descriptions, standardized procedures, and other guidelines for employees and managers.

Process is more dynamic, fluid, and responsive to inputs of information and energy. It is somewhat analogous to the physiologic activities of the human body which occur continuously as the systems within the body make adaptations in an effort to maintain balance. Process in an organizational system is probably best exemplified by such managerial activities as communicating, leading, interacting with people, making decisions, and seeking solutions to problems.

THE HUMAN RELATIONS ERA

One of the earliest, best known, and most controversial studies of people at work was made by a group of researchers from the Harvard Business School at the Hawthorne Works of Western Electric near Chicago. These studies are known as the Hawthorne studies; their impact on motivation theory and management practice continues to be felt up to the present. Criticisms of the research methods used and the ethical dimensions of the manner in which the results were interpreted do not alter the fact that the Hawthorne studies ushered in a new and exciting period in the evolution of management thought. Although there have been conflicting interpretations of the findings of these studies, there is general agreement that they laid the groundwork for intensive interest in and continued study of human relationships in an organizational setting.

Motivation theory and its application to the practice of management will be discussed in more detail in Chapter 6 where the details of the Hawthorne studies are presented more fully. For the present we will turn to the work of Douglas McGregor and his conclusions about relationships between one's philosophy about the nature of man and his/her preference for a particular style of management.

McGregor's theory X and theory Y

Recognizing that people often have firmly entrenched ideas about whether humans are inherently evil or inherently good, McGregor concluded that management style depends on the manager's philosophy of human nature and his/her beliefs about how people feel about work.

According to McGregor, reductive assumptions (Theory X) produce a strict, authoritarian style of management that is the least effective in motivating others. At the opposite extreme (Theory Y), developmental assumptions lead to a liberal style of management that is more effective. The two sets of assumptions are as follows:

theory X assumptions

- The average human being has an inherent dislike of work and will avoid it if he can.

- Because of this characteristic, most people must be coerced, controlled, directed, and threatened with punishment to get them to put forth the effort needed to achieve organizational objectives.

- The average human being prefers to be directed, wishes to avoid responsibility, has relatively little ambition, and wants security above all.

theory Y assumptions

- The expenditure of physical and mental effort in work is as natural as play or rest.

- External control and the threat of punishment are not the only means of bringing about effort toward organizational objectives. Man will exercise self-direction and self-control in the service of objectives to which he is committed.

- Commitment to objectives is a function of the rewards associated with their achievement.

- The average human being learns under proper conditions not only to accept, but also to seek, responsibility.

- The capacity to exercise a high degree of imagination, ingenuity and creativity in the solution of organizational problems is widely, not narrowly, distributed in the population.

- Under the conditions of modern industrial life the intellectual potentialities of the average human being are only partially utilized.[8]

McGregor's work is based on Maslow's hierarchy of human needs theory. It is his contention that by meeting the higher as well as the lower levels of human need the managers of organizations are better able to integrate the goals of the organization with the personal goals of its employees. He identified the "essential task of management" as a process in which managers create a working environment that (1) creates opportunities for personal growth; (2) allows for the release of human potential; and (3) provides guidance for the achievement of both personal and organizational goals.[9]

Figure 1.3 presents a self-test to determine your own assumptions about people and the kind of guidance you think they need to assure efficient and effective delivery of patient care. The self-test is not a measurement of your ability to be a good or bad manager; it is intended only as a kind of self-analysis to increase your awareness of your thoughts and feelings about the people with whom you work. The items on the self-test are derived from the work of M. Scott Myers[10] and David Kolb, et al.[11]

figure 1.3   self-test on assumptions about people

DIRECTIONS: There are ten *paired* statements. Each pair is a set. In the space provided at the end of each pair, place a rating using a scale of 1 to 10. Notice that the *total rating* for each pair must equal 10. A rating of 0 for one of the pair would indicate that you do not agree with the statement at all. A rating of 10 for one of the statements would indicate that you are in total agreement.

1. It is only human to avoid work if you possibly can. (a) __
    *People usually avoid work because their work has (b) __
    no meaning for them. (10)

2. If employees are helped to learn more about the (c) __
    tasks they are expected to perform, they will have a
    better attitude toward their work.
    *It is dangerous to give subordinates too much in- (d) __
    formation because they may try to do something (10)
    that would be harmful to a patient.

3. Seeking input from subordinates is not worth the (e) __
    time and effort because most health care workers
    at this level cannot provide much useful informa-
    tion.
    *Asking subordinates for their ideas and sugges- (f) __
    tions broadens their perspective and also in- (10)
    creases the possibility that acceptable solutions
    to problems will be found.

4. If people aren't very creative or imaginative in (g) __
    solving patient care problems, it's probably
    because so few people have these talents.
    *The capacity to be creative and imaginative is a (h) __
    relatively common human characteristic, and if (10)
    people don't use much ingenuity and imagination
    it is probably because supervisory styles and atti-
    tudes are stifling.

figure 1.3 cont'd

5.   People tend to raise their standards if they are (i)   —
     held accountable for their own behavior and for
     correcting their mistakes.
     *People tend to lower their standards if they are (j)   —
     not punished for unacceptable behavior and mis-   (10)
     takes.

6.   Most people would rather be told what to do than (k)   —
     have to set their own objectives.
     *Most people will achieve objectives more enthu- (l)   —
     siastically if they have participated in formulating   (10)
     them and are committed to their achievement.

7.   A nurse-manager must be respected; therefore it (m)   —
     weakens her prestige to admit that a subordinate
     was right and she was wrong.
     *Because workers at all levels should be respected (n)   —
     equally, a nurse-manager's prestige can be   (10)
     strengthened by admitting that a subordinate was
     right and she was wrong.

8.   Most people are more concerned about making (o)   —
     enough money than they are about such in-
     tangibles as responsibility and recognition.
     *If people are provided with challenging work that (p)   —
     is interesting and gives them a sense of ac-   (10)
     complishment, they will be less concerned about
     such things as salary and fringe benefits.

9.   If health care workers are allowed to participate in (q)   —
     setting their own standards of performance, they
     tend to set them higher than supervisors would.
     *If healthcare workers are allowed to participate in (r)   —
     setting their own standards of performance, they   (10)
     would tend to set them lower than supervisors
     would.

10. As a worker's knowledge about and freedom to (s)   —
     carry out his job increases, he needs more external
     controls to keep him in line.
     *As a worker's knowledge about and freedom to (t)   —
     carry out his job increases there is less need to   (10)
     exert control to insure satisfactory performance.

figure 1.3 cont'd

Scoring:

To determine your score on the X-Y Scale, add up the points you assigned to the following:

Theory X score = sum of (a), (d), (e), (g), (j), (l), (m), (o), (r), & (s).

Theory Y score = sum of (b), (c), (f), (h), (i), (k), (n), (p), (q), & (t).

The sum of the numbers you assigned to each statement should tell you how closely you associate with either Theory X or Theory Y. Complete agreement with the theory would be a score of 100.

---

participative management

The writings of McGregor and other humanists have made important contributions to the development of the concept of participative management, that is, the notion that management is a cooperative effort in which the subordinates take an active part in all of the functional activities once considered to be the exclusive domain of administration.

It should be made clear from the outset that participative management is not a valid approach to all of managerial problems in every kind of situation. The degree to which an individual or group of employees are able to participate in the management process depends on the kind of decisions that must be made, the problems being confronted, and the time, effort, and competencies needed to take an active part in these activities.

Participative management is by its very nature a group effort. Although it may mean that at times a manager sits down with a subordinate to formulate personal objectives for the employee's growth in his/her job, these objectives cannot be at odds with the objectives of the patient care unit and the goals of the organization.

There must be mutual trust and respect among all parties and a willingness to be open and direct in their dealings with one another. Good communication is essential. Without it there cannot be the give and take that any cooperative and integrated effort must have.

Additionally, participative management demands careful planning and close attention to details. Participants must be willing to invest time and energy, particularly in the early phases of the process. It also is important that they take the long view, realizing that the achievement of short-term objectives will lead to larger long-term goals. For example, employees who work hard at identifying a specific problem, planning for its resolution, and taking part in implementing and evaluating *their* plans will develop their own skills and potential for growth. Having someone else solve problems and make decisions might be the most expedient and least painful way to deal with the situation but it also fosters dependence and irresponsibility that in the long run will be harmful to them and the organization.

In order to keep conflict at a tolerable and manageable level, it is important that participants reach some agreement about what is important, valuable, and worth striving for. Interpersonal skills and the ability to get people to work together as a group are necessary for successful utilization of this approach. Leaders also should be particularly adept at clarifying objectives and measuring progress toward their achievement. Management by Objectives (MBO), which we will discuss in the following pages, is a valuable system of management techniques for implementing the concept of participative management.

management by objectives

Peter Drucker, an economist, and one of the most prolific writers in the field of management, is credited with coining the phrase *management by objectives* in his classic work published in 1956 under the title *The Practice of Management.* Management by objectives (MBO) is essentially a structural concept rather than one of process. It contributes to the skeletal framework or the more stable components of the management process, particularly those functions concerned with planning and control. Its emphasis is on performance and outcome rather than input, and on self-control and self-direction rather than supervisor control and enforced effectiveness. It can be an invaluable system of techniques for the first-line manager because it encourages decentralization of authority and responsibility and provides guidelines by which first-line managers and subordinates can decide what their objectives are and how they want to achieve them.

The basic techniques of MBO include the development of measurable goals at all levels within the organization; the participation of employees in determining standards of performance and expected outcomes; and periodic evaluation and appraisal to determine progress toward the accomplishment of goals.

In this context goals and objectives have roughly the same meaning and often are used interchangeably by many authors. Some use the term *objectives* in a more general sense and in reference to long-term results and overall purposes. Others use the word *goal* to designate these desired ends and the word *objective* to indicate more immediate and short-term goals. There are at least three general types of goals or objectives:

- The overall mission and goals of the organization as a whole; for example, the goal of providing certain kinds of health care services to a community.

- Department and unit objectives, as for example those of the Nursing Department and such patient care units as ICU, Pediatrics, and Medical and Surgical units. These are also called *performance* objectives.

- The personal development or career goals of individuals; for example a staff nurse's objectives for improvement in knowledge and skills and the development of her potential for growth.

We can see that there is ample opportunity for conflict in the development of goals at the organizational, departmental, unit, and individual levels. This potential for conflict among groups and individuals should not be underestimated. Ideally, the goals and the means by which they will be achieved are compatible and mutually supporting at all levels. In reality, they oftentimes are in conflict and diminish the chances for a concerted effort to meet the needs of the patients and clients the organization and its employees purport to serve. The management of conflict is discussed in Chapter 9.

Most hospitals, clinics, and other kinds of health care organizations have adopted some form of MBO. If you are not familiar with the mission, purposes, and goals of the organization in which you work, you should obtain a copy, read it thoroughly, and keep it on file. Objectives for the Nursing Department also should be written and readily accessible to first-line managers and employees. If the administration of the organization is committed to the principles of participative management and MBO, supervisors and head nurses will have opportunity to take part in developing and periodically revising departmental and unit objectives.

Professional nurses are fortunate in having excellent guidelines from the American Nurses Association and the National League for Nursing, which are helpful in formulating departmental and unit objectives. These standards of nursing practice and nursing services also are helpful in setting personal career goals for managers and staff nurses.

If you want to use MBO techniques for planning and evaluating work performance on your own patient care unit you must be realistic about what it can and cannot do for you and for those who work under your direction. Management by objectives does not necessarily need to be employed throughout the entire organizational system in order for you to use the techniques on your unit. However your objectives for the unit and for individual employees cannot be incompatible with the mission, philosophy, and objectives or goals of the organization and nursing department.

writing objectives

The previous discussion of MBO is a greatly oversimplified explanation of a many-faceted concept. If you expect to take part in an MBO program and carry out its techniques you should receive instruction during an inservice education program or a workshop conducted by consultants who have expertise in this aspect of management. There is always the possibility that these will not be readily available to you. When such is the case and you still want to utilize this system for planning and controlling activities on your unit, you can take the initiative and set up a self-directed course of study. The references and suggested readings at the end of this chapter can be a starting point for you. One of the major reasons why MBO doesn't work in an organization is that supervisors and head nurses are not adequately prepared to accept responsibility for participating in the program.

Another cause of failure of MBO is the inability of personnel to write clear, concise, and easily understood objectives. Volumes have been written about how to state objectives. So much, in fact, that the novice is easily intimidated and discouraged. One step you might take to overcome this problem is to establish some priorities. Prepare a roughly drawn list of things you would like to see accomplished and then classify them as: (1) *critical* objectives that must be met, (2) *necessary* objectives that should be met, and (3) *desirable* objectives that need to be met, perhaps sometime in the future.

A clearly written and concise objective is one written in plain language and least likely to be misinterpreted by the reader. For example, if you intend to change your staffing pattern and assignment system so that the work load on your units is more evenly distributed, then say so. If you intend to eventually get a ward secretary to handle paper work and free your nursing staff for clinical nursing duties, again, say so. Objectives evolve as you work on them. The more thought given to what you really want to accomplish, the more explicit you will be in stating your objectives.

Other considerations in the writing of objectives are the consequences resulting from implementation of your planned objectives. First, are you talking about an objective for the future that maintains the status quo of a nursing task, or are you planning a change with the hope that it will improve the situation? The first is a *functional objective*. The task—for example, monitoring the I.V. fluids on all patients—is routinely carried out, but you want to document this function, setting standards for carrying it out.

The second type, in which improvement is the aim, is a *change objective*. For example, equipment and supplies on your unit are taking wing and flying away; charge slips are not to be found for materials used and shelves are not being restocked. Your objective is to institute a system so that the mystery of the empty shelves is solved.

Every objective that is intended to be explicit, task-oriented, and focused on expected results should contain the following elements:

- *Who* will perform the task?
- *What* will be done?
- *How well* will it be done?
- *When* will it be done?
- *Where* will it be done?
- What will it *cost*? (if pertinent)

Writing clearly defined objectives comes with practice. It forces you to think through the situation at hand and consider all the factors that might influence the successful accomplishment of a specific goal. Above all, you must discipline yourself to put your objectives *in writing*. Whatever you and the members of your staff hope to accomplish, it is unlikely that you will ever attain your goals if you keep them in your head and discuss them occasionally with the hope that some day they will become realities. Management by objectives can help you shift from crisis management and firefighting to a more systematic approach that utilizes carefully thought out and mutually agreed upon objectives.

One of the major difficulties in writing objectives is deciding how specific to be. Should the objective specify every detail of a plan or can it be a more general guide? There is no satisfactory answer to that question. It depends on your purpose for writing the objective, whom it will affect, how well you know the persons to be affected, and how the objective will be used. Only you and the members of the group know what your needs are.

If you set up an objective that requires a change, everyone involved must know the specifics of the change. The *how* component of the objective may require *subobjectives* that will enable every one to reach the major objective. Your objective might be that everyone under your direction will use a particular system for insuring that the emergency cart is always fully stocked. Your subobjectives would give the details of the system so that everyone can use it effectively. Perhaps everyone knows the system, but it will not work if you assume that they all know it and, in fact, there are some who do not.

examples of written objectives

Some sample objectives are presented below. Check each one to see if you think it meets the criteria of who, what, where, when, how well, and how costly.

- *Objective for the head nurse in a long-term care facility.*
  Institute the SOAP system for charting progress notes on all patients in the West wing, from April 1 to April 30, with 100 percent accuracy as measured according to the outlined procedure taught to all nursing personnel on that unit, at a cost not to exceed the present cost for charting.

- *Objective for team leader responsible for one LPN and two nursing assistants.*
  Continue to hold a 15-minute conference with all team members on duty, at or near 11:00 a.m. on Tuesdays and Fridays of each week for the purpose of reviewing patient care assignment and revising them according to the decisions of the group.

- *Objective for a charge nurse, 11-7 shift, 60-bed surgical floor.*
  Prepare by the end of this week a list of duties unique to the night shift as a first step in a plan for orienting new graduates assigned to night duty on this unit.

- *Team members, 3-11 shift, 48-bed medical unit.*
  Institute by next Monday our new system for recording I&O in each patient's room at the time it is measured, for a trial period of two weeks, and with 100 percent success in having an I&O record for every patient at the end of our shift each night.

  Subobjective: Each person on the team will have demonstrated to another team member the ability to use the new system,

  or

  Subobjective: Between now and next Monday each team member will have demonstrated to the satisfaction of another team member the ability to use the new system and an explanation of its purpose.

THE SYSTEMS APPROACH AND CONTINGENCY MANAGEMENT

As explained earlier, the proliferation of information from a variety of disciplines has greatly enhanced the body of knowledge known as organization theory, but it has made it extremely difficult to deal with the topic as a unified whole. This is true of many of the older, better established fields of study as well as the newcomers. In trying to make it easier for scientists to interact with and learn from one another, an attempt was made to develop a theory that would integrate knowledge from all of the disciplines.

General Systems Theory (GST) is a concept pioneered by Ludwig Von Bertalanffy. It provides a theoretical framework for identifying general relationships in the real world. The modern systems approach to management views the organization as an open, sociotechnical system.

A system may be defined as an entity that behaves in certain ways because of interactions between and among its individual parts or subsystems. An *open* system is one that interacts with the objects in its environment. The characteristics or properties common to all systems are *structure* (being), *function* (behaving), and *evolution* (becoming).[12] A system can be a human person or some other biologic entity, a group of people, a technological entity such as a heating and air-conditioning system, or an organization such as a hospital or clinic.

If one considers an organization such as a hospital or community health center as a system, then the *structure* of the system would be composed of organizational charts, rules, policies, and other evidence previously mentioned when we discussed structure and process.

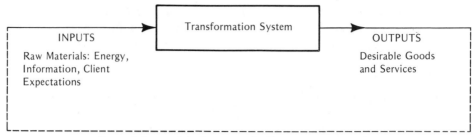

figure 1.4   model of an organization as an open system

The *functions* or *behaving* characteristics of a system are the things that are done to maintain the integrity of its structure, transform inputs into outputs, and respond to stimuli from objects in the internal and external environment. The human body performs many functions to maintain its structural integrity, to transform nutrients and oxygen into energy and cellular materials into growth and repair, to eliminate waste, and to adapt to its environment both internal (body fluids) and external. An organization also maintains its structure, but in slightly different ways. It enforces rules, policies, and other elements in its structural framework. It utilizes the input of human and material resources energy and information, transforming them into the output of products or services to the people who use them. (See Figure 1.4.)

Later, when we discuss change, we will go into more detail about the environments in which organizational systems operate and the relationship between environmental forces and change. Since viable organizational systems must change with time, the *becoming* aspect of a system refers to the changes, adaptations, and adjustments that a system must make if it is to survive.

The concepts of general systems theory (GST) are certainly not simple, and it is not my intention to convey the impression that they can be learned with ease. However, the notion of adaptation, equilibrium, homeostasis, and positive and negative feedback should be familiar to you. They are incorporated into current writings on human physiology, the health-illness continuum, and the role of the nurse in preventing disease and maintaining health through the nursing process. The transfer of these concepts into the field of management should not be too difficult. Remember, the major purpose of GST is to establish some means by which philosophers, behavioral scientists, physicists, nurses, managers, and a host of others can talk with one another and be fairly well understood.

contingency management

A contingency is a possibility, a condition. Contingency management is based on the belief that the most effective way to practice management is to take into consideration all the conditions existing in a particular management situation and to choose managerial styles and techniques most suitable for these conditions. Earlier theorists believed that there is a general theory of management and basic principles and practices that could be applied to any situation to resolve the problems of management. Contingency management theorists refute that belief. They contend that there is no one best way to manage. Rather, many variables in the situation dictate the way in which the problem should be handled, for example, the nature of the specific task to be done, the kind of people performing the task, or the resources available.

As a professional nurse, you have used the contingency approach in the management of nursing care. Your plans are based on the individual needs of the patient and then implemented according to resources available and the patient's response to the plan. The kind of nursing care that is prescribed and administered depends on the conditions of the situation. In other words, it is conditional or situational.

Contingency management in nursing requires an in-depth knowledge of nursing theory and practice. Contingency management in an organization also requires in-depth knowledge and special skills. One must be adept in interpersonal relationships, have facility in communication, and some ability to be flexible—able to use more than one style of leadership. According to contingency theorists, an effective leader is one who can act in different ways to meet changing conditions. In some instances an authoritarian style may be most appropriate while another situation may call for application of the principles of participative management and a more democratic style of leadership.

Throughout the remainder of this text we will emphasize the contingency approach to management. It is hoped that you will gain insight into your own attitudes and preferences, your abilities and needs for improvement in knowledge and skills, and the importance of fitting the approach to a problem to the conditions under which the problem is manifested.

REFERENCES

[1] R. A. MacKenzie, "The management process in 3 D," *Harvard Business Review*, (Nov.-Dec., 1969), Reprinted with permission in *Journal of Nursing Administration*, (Nov., 1979), p. 30.

[2] J. H. Donnelly, Jr., et al, *Fundamentals of Management: Functions, Behaviors, Models*, (Austin, Tex.: Business Publications, Inc., 1971).

[3] MacKenzie, *op. cit.*

[4] F. W. Taylor, "The principles of scientific management," *Scientific Man.* (New York: Harper and Row, Inc., 1947), p. 83.

[5]C. S. George, Jr., *The History of Management Thought*, (Englewood Cliffs, N.J.: Prentice-Hall, 1972).

[6]C. Schmalenberg and M. Kramer, "Dreams and reality: Where do they meet?," *Journal of Nursing Administration*, (Oct., 1976), p. 35.

[7]C. S. George, *op. cit.*

[8]D. McGregor, *Leadership and Motivation*, (Cambridge, Mass.: The M.I.T. Press, 1966).

[9]D. McGregor, *The Human Side of Enterprise*, (New York: McGraw-Hill Co., 1960).

[10]M. Scott Myers, *Every Employee a Manager*, (New York: McGraw-Hill Co., 1970).

[11]David Kolb, et al, *Organizational Psychology: An Experimental Approach*, 2nd ed., (Englewood Cliffs, N.J.: Prentice-Hall, Inc., 1974).

[12]H. R. Bobbitt, Jr., et al, *Organizational Behavior*, (Englewood Cliffs, N.J.: Prentice-Hall, Inc., 1974).

SUGGESTED READINGS

M. H. Cantor, "Philosophy, purpose and objectives: Why do we have them?" *The Techniques of Management*, (Wakefield, Mass.: Contemporary Publishing Co., 1975), p. 9.

R. B. Fine, "Application of leadership theory," *The Nursing Clinics of North America*, 13:1. (Philadelphia: W. B. Saunders Co., 1978), p. 139.

H. Gassett, "Participative planned change," *Supervisor Nurse*, (March, 1976), p. 34.

A. Gerstenfeld, "MBO revisited: Focus on health systems," *Health Care Management Review*, (Fall, 1977), p. 51.

P. Hersey. K. H. Blanchard, and E. LaMonica, "A situational approach to leadership," *Supervisor Nurse*, (May, 1976), p. 17.

B. S. Hill, "Participative management: A valid alternative to traditional organizational behavior," *Supervisor Nurse*, (March, 1976), p. 19.

P. W. Miller, "Open minds to new ideas: An injunction for nursing leaders." *Supervisor Nurse*, (April, 1976). p. 18.

P. Niessner, "Participative management in the ICU," *Supervisor Nurse*, (March, 1978), p. 41.

J. Palmer, "Management by objectives," *Journal of Nursing Administration*, (Sept./Oct., 1973).

L. Shores, "Staff development for leadership," *The Nursing Clinics of North America*, 13:1, (Philadelphia: W. B. Saunders Co., 1978), p. 103.

chapter 2
index

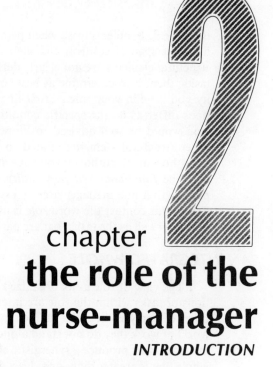

chapter
the role of the nurse-manager
INTRODUCTION

A role is a complex set of expectations, values and norms; the concept of role is concerned with thoughts, perceptions, and actions.[1] From these various mental and physical activities people develop their expectations about those who act out or fulfill a role. Social scientists define a role as *a set of organized behaviors that are associated with a given social position.* For example, the position of first-line manager brings with it status and certain expectations about how the person in such a position should behave. These expectations arise from within the individual in the role and from people and other elements in his/her environment. As might be expected, there often is conflict arising from differences in the expectations that these various individuals have and the values on which their expectations are based.

However, our concern in this chapter will not be with the kinds of role conflict that can occur, but rather with helping you develop some of your own expectations about the role of first-line manager. Role conflicts are important, and they will be discussed more fully in Chapter 9; for the present you will need to decide what your role should be and how you can perform in that role. The accuracy with which you perceive your role, and the skill with which you can perform the tasks within it will have a definite impact on your ability to carry out your duties and responsibilities efficiently and effectively.[2]

Role expectations for an individual who is part of an organizational system are not carried out in a vacuum but within the structural matrix of the system. Problems arise when people do not understand lines of authority, their span of control, and their areas of responsibility, or when these structural elements are not clearly defined and communicated.[3] One of your tasks, then, is to determine as best you can what authority and responsibility you have in your role as first-line manager. The structure of organizations differ as do the specific conditions or situations in the organization. You would be well advised to know the policies, rules, regulations, and other structural elements related to your position, and you will need to know how much authority you have in enforcing them.

The *functional* and *personality requirements* for the part you are to play as first-line manager are the essence of this chapter. You will notice that in this context the word *role* is used to indicate the whole-task concept of role as well as the tasks that are part of the whole.

AN INTEGRATED WHOLE

The view of role as an organized set of behaviors implies that the functions or tasks within the role are interrelated and interdependent. For purposes of analysis the tasks can be separated and scrutinized, but in the real world of work they do not stand alone. Peter Drucker says that the effective manager must produce a synergistic effect; that is, he/she must create a true whole that is greater than, or at least different from, the sum of its parts.[4]

Another researcher, Leonard Sayles, has systematically studied the role of the manager, and analyzed the job to determine the tasks that make up the observable whole. In his words, the manager is:

> like a symphony orchestra conductor, endeavoring to maintain a melodious performance in which the contributions of the various instruments are coordinated and sequenced, patterned and paced, while the orchestra members are having various personal difficulties, stage hands are moving music stands, alternating excessive heat and cold are creating audience and instrument problems, and the sponsor of the concert is insisting on irrational changes in the program.[5]

Now, let's change the scene to the patient care setting, paraphrasing Dr. Sayles' description of the job of the manager.

> The nurse-manager must orchestrate total patient care in which the contributions of the personnel from the various hospital departments are coordinated and sequenced, patterned and paced, so that the patient is neither exhausted from too much attention nor neglected by too little. During a rapidly moving series of events the available stock of supplies and equipment is being depleted, some patients are in need of immediate attention while others are being admitted to the unit, anxious family members are hovering about, the physicians are writing new orders, and the nursing supervisor is insisting that revisions of objectives for the patient care unit be in her office no later than this afternoon.

The scene described above is probably all too familiar to anyone who has been in charge of a patient care unit on a typical working day. In fact, it is not unlike the work day of any first-line manager, regardless of the setting, the services provided, or the product produced. Research studies have repeatedly shown that a first-line manager's work life is hectic and challenging. And yet the work gets done, progress is made, and objectives are met. This is possible because there has been behind-the-scenes planning, organizing, and controlling. To be more specific, the manager has been performing a variety of related tasks and functions that are appropriate to his/her role.

In the following pages we will attempt to break down the whole-task role of the first-line manager into some of its more critical parts. No claim is made as to the completeness of the list. It is, however, a start, a beginning point for self-evaluation and self-direction in the fulfillment of your role. Hunt defines *role conception* as the individual's *idealized* version of the part he/she should play, and *role performance* as the individual's actual behavior.[6] Once you have a conception of how you should behave, you will be better able to measure your performance and set realistic goals for improvement.

ANALYSIS OF THE ROLE OF MANAGER

Systematic research studies of managers at work turn up some interesting data about what managers do and how they spend their time during a work day. From his analysis of the manager's job and his subsequent synthesis of the tasks of management, Mintzberg derived ten major roles. In his view, the formal authority and status or position of the manager gives rise to three sets of roles: interpersonal, informational, and decisional. Figure 2.1 shows the relationships among the sets; that is, the interpersonal roles give rise to informational roles, which in turn enable the manager to play decisional roles.[7]

figure 2.1   relationships among sets of roles; from Mintzberg's ten major roles
Reprinted by permission of the Harvard Business Review. Exhibit/Excerpt from "The Manager's job: folklore and fact" by Henry Mintzberg (July-August 1975). Copyright © 1975 by the President and Fellows of Harvard College; all rights reserved.

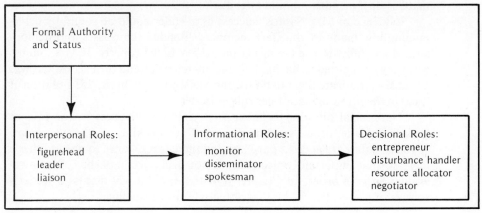

The six roles discussed in the following pages are the result of an attempt to apply to the nurse-manager's role the concepts explored by Mintzberg and others. If you have the time and inclination, you might conduct some informal research of your own and develop a list of behavioral roles from observations and interviews with head nurses and other first-line managers in health care organizations.

as leader

One of the first roles to come to mind when considering the duties of the nurse in charge is that of leader. In this role you are expected to identify problems, delegate tasks, effect change, and motivate your subordinates. As a leader you recognize the individual needs, talents, and abilities of each employee and attempt to reconcile your employees' personal goals with those of the agency.

Occupying the position of manager does not automatically make a person a leader. Management and leadership are not synonymous. A manager can be said to function as a leader only when there is evidence that those who work under his/her direction are behaving in a certain way because of his/her influence on them. There also must be evidence that both the leader and the led are working to accomplish the same objectives. A manager could hardly be called a leader if he/she is headed in one direction while the troops are either marching off in pursuit of another goal or aimlessly milling about.

An example of evidence of leadership can be found in the area of decision making. Consider the following: Maria Santos is a head nurse on a surgical ward. Her supervisor has told her that Central Supply recently bought some new gastric suction machines that are more efficient than the older models presently in use, but the new models are a bit trickier to operate. Mrs. Santos learns that in-service education classes will be held for employees who need instruction in the use of the new machines. She decides that her staff members should attend.

Evidence of Mrs. Santos' success as a leader could be found by determining how many of the staff members attended the classes and demonstrated an ability to use the newer model machine properly. If Mrs. Santos was truly committed to having her staff members attend the classes, but was not able to motivate them to do so, she was unsuccessful (in this situation at least) in the performance of her role as leader.

The crucial question in measuring your effectiveness in the role of leader is whether or not you and your staff are working together as a team. If you and they are at cross purposes and there is resistance to one another's ideas so that important objectives are not being accomplished, then a reevaluation is in order. In Chapter 6 of this text we will discuss a leader's sources of power, that is, his/her potential for influencing others.

as liaison person

Nurse managers who are, in fact, integrators of patient care must somehow coordinate the activities of other health care providers so that each patient can benefit from their services. In the liaison role you must deal with your counterparts in other departments of the health care facility, as well as with the staff of outside health-related agencies. One of the greatest needs of a client inside or outside a health care facility is help in getting a complex health care delivery system to focus on his case and do for him what it is supposed to do.[8]

Perhaps we should pause here and clarify what we mean by *patient care.* In the context of this discussion, *medical care* includes the medical treatments, surgical procedures, diagnostic tests and other events that are specifically ordered by the physician. *Nursing care* refers to measures taken by a nurse in an effort to prevent, alleviate, or resolve the problems considered to be amenable to actions that are within the realm of nursing practice. *Patient care* encompasses all of the preventive, diagnostic and therapeutic activities that are provided by members of a health care team striving to meet the patient's individual needs. Patient care is the outcome of collaboration, consultation, and cooperation among the team members within the structure of an organizational system and the larger health care system.

In your liaison role you establish contact with your peers for purposes of providing, receiving, clarifying and acting on information about patient care, or requesting specific services for the patient and his family. Whereas most of your activities in other roles are directed vertically upward to superiors and downward to subordinates, as liaison you direct your activities laterally. In this role the successful nurse-manager behaves in an assertive manner, dealing with other members of the health care team as a member, not as captain nor as water boy.

A nurse-manager's success in the liaison role must begin with a perception of herself as a professional who is an expert in her own field. While she is responsible for seeing to it that the prescribed medical regimen is carried out as intended by the physician, she does not blindly follow his orders. She confers with the physician as a colleague and keeps him informed of the patient's response to the total patient care plan.

Some agencies employ non-nurse *unit managers* to lighten the nurse-manager's load of administrative duties that are not directly related to the nursing care of patients. Problems with this approach to unit management occur when there is no clear distinction made between nursing and non-nursing tasks. Areas of responsibility overlap, efforts are duplicated, and some tasks rest in limbo, unclaimed by either the unit manager or the nurse-manager. In spite of these difficulties non-nurse unit managers have been used successfully in hospitals and clinics that have planned carefully before initiating the program and prepared the nursing staff and unit managers thoroughly before putting the plan into action. Full utilization of a unit manager is possible if there is a cooperative effort between the nurse-manager and the unit manager and mutual respect for the contributions each can make toward achievement of common goals.

A brief discussion of non-nurse unit managers is appropriate here because many of the tasks performed within the liaison role can be done by someone other than a nurse as long as that person has a sound understanding of the whole health care system. If you are a nurse-manager in an institution or agency that employs non-nurse unit managers, you can be relieved of some of the time-consuming tasks that are more desk oriented than patient oriented. It is not realistic however, to think that a non-nurse unit manager can relieve the nurse-manager of all non-nursing activities. Unit managers can influence the efficiency and improve the caliber of service provided to clients and patients, but they really cannot completely free the nurse to nurse.[9]

If you do not have a non-nurse unit manager working in your unit, you can delegate many non-nursing tasks to a well-trained ward clerk or secretary working under your supervision. This arrangement is more easily handled because the lines of authority and areas of responsibility can be more clearly defined.

as evaluator

Assessment of the quality and quantity of work done by an organizational group is an essential task of the first-line manager. Evaluations, critical appraisals, and on-the-spot judgments are intuitively made by any person who accepts responsibility for a particular situation. Evaluation is a natural and ongoing activity that takes place consciously or unconsciously in the mind of a manager.

In contrast to this rather casual and disorganized way of forming evaluations, there is a systematic and more formalized kind of appraisal that is closely related to, if not synonymous with, the controlling aspects of management. Systematic evaluation by a first-line manager is carried out for the purpose of determining the efficiency of resources and their effectiveness in meeting goals and objectives. A systematic program of evaluation is interrelated with planning, organizing, staffing, and directing, as well as controlling.

Among the resources to be evaluated by the first-line manager are the material resources needed to get the work done. Later, when we discuss the nurse-manager's role as allocator of resources, we will see that evaluation is a component of this role. Equipment and supplies that are not cost effective should be replaced by those that are. Space that is not being used efficiently and effectively can be reassigned so that it serves more useful purposes.

The appraisal of employee performance is resisted by many first-line managers because historically it has been done for purposes of conferring extrinsic rewards and punishment. On the basis of merit ratings people were given wage increases, promotions, demotions, and notice of suspension or firing. Highly subjective evaluations that rate personality and personal characteristics, rather than measurable performance behaviors, are recognized as being a threat to an employee's self-esteem and personal security. [10]

In Chapter 10 of this text we will discuss employee appraisal and the newer trends toward evaluation of performance in terms of results or outcomes. A more humanistic approach emphasizes the achievement of personal goals, development of potential, and progress toward meeting higher levels of human needs. The manager functions more as counselor and guide than as judge and jury.

It is suggested by some researchers that goal-oriented evaluation of professional and technical nursing personnel can help reduce turnover rates and serve as a tool for the retention of competent personnel. [11, 12]

Yura and Walsh suggest that the nurse-manager should begin with herself in her role as evaluator of personnel. [13] Knowledge of her own strengths and weaknesses, values, interests, and aptitudes can be helpful in identifying and evaluating specific competencies in others. As a manager develops insight into her own progress toward personal objectives, she becomes more confident in her ability to appraise and guide the growth and development of her subordinates.

In her role as evaluator, the first-line manager should be aware that her own competence is being evaluated continuously and informally by her subordinates. Moore and Simendinger point out that formal and systematic evaluations are almost always conducted from the top down. A broader and more constructive concept of evaluation would, they suggest, allow subordinates to express their view of their immediate supervisor's job performance in a more formal and confidential manner. Among the items listed on their sample subordinate-superior rating form are such characteristics as responsibility, honesty, leadership ability, concern for others, and self-discipline. [14]

Tasks within the role of evaluator might be summarized as follows:

- Appraisal of existing material resources and those under consideration for future use.

- Establishment of personal goals and objectives for professional growth of the manager herself and for her subordinates. Determination of criteria and standards by which specific characteristics and behaviors can be measured.

- Use of evaluation tools and techniques for measurement of traits and behaviors, including the printed appraisal forms required by the organization.

as teacher and developer of resources

If one accepts the concept of management as the development of people, then it follows that a most important managerial role would be that of teacher. Much of what a nurse-manager's subordinates learn is taught to them by her example. This is a powerful teaching technique, but it is an informal, generalized way of teaching that does not always recognize the individual learning needs of employees. In order to develop the potential of each staff member and improve her performance a more formal kind of education must take place. Both informal and formal must, however, be ongoing.

Activities within the teacher role must be planned and purposeful. They should include assessment of learning needs, preparation of learning objectives in behavioral terms, planning appropriate teaching-learning activities, implementing the plan and evaluating its effectiveness.

The learning needs of an employee can be determined by observing her at work and talking with her about the particular aspects of patient care that are confusing, frightening, or in some way difficult for her to perform with confidence. Fulfillment of the teaching role need not be complicated and highly structured. Helping an employee to learn a procedure correctly and safely or to understand new concepts and techniques can be as satisfying to the teacher as to the learner. It is a good investment of time and energy because of the long-term gains in peace of mind and time saved. The better informed and more competent employee reduces the risks inherent in delegation and gives the manager more freedom to assign to others which she might otherwise have to perform herself.

Here is an example of a "mini lesson" in which the nurse-manager demonstrates fulfillment of the role of teacher and developer of potential.

Mr. Long has been employed only recently as charge nurse for one wing of a long-term care facility. One evening he overheard two nursing attendants discussing the mental confusion exhibited by some of their patients. The attendants seemed to be saying that the best way to handle these patients is to agree with whatever they are saying, right or wrong. They apparently were not aware of the techniques and benefits of reality therapy in the management of disoriented and confused patients.

Mr. Long asked the nursing attendants if they had ever heard of reality therapy and they replied that they had not. The attendants expressed an interest in learning more about it. Plans were made to obtain some readings on the topic and have some discussion of the concept. During the discussion plans for utilizing some of the techniques were finalized.

After three meetings lasting about twenty minutes each, the nursing attendants were prepared to put into practice what they had learned. One month later another meeting was held and the nursing attendants reported that their techniques were helpful in reorienting the patients and they intended to continue using them.

Most larger hospitals and health care agencies have a department of in-service education or staff development that is responsible for orientation of new personnel and education of employees in regard to policies, procedures, and use of new equipment. The programs of departments of this kind do not, however, relieve the nurse-manager of her responsibilities in the role of teacher. The in-service education classes may supplement the ongoing teaching activities that should take place on the patients' care unit, but they are not a substitute for them.

The roles of evaluator and teacher are so closely interwoven it is almost impossible to discuss one without touching on the other. Both are essential to the notion that a manager's primary task is to help employees meet their needs for esteem and personal growth. So essential, in fact, that each topic will be covered in depth in later chapters of this text.

as allocator of resources

An effective manager is aware of the resources available to her and utilizes these resources appropriately. The major categories of resources are time, money, and people. Not one of these resources is unlimited; there are just so many hours in the day, so much money in the budget, and so many employees for staffing a unit. The success of a nurse-manager is directly related to her ability to work within the constraints of time, money, and staff.

time

We will begin with the resource of time, which is always in very short supply in the life of every busy and productive person. A good manager takes control of her time and uses it to fullest advantage. Rather than resent the almost constant demands on her time, she sets priorities on and limits her responses to those demands that are most important. She then makes the most of the time that she must spend with others.

If for example, it is part of the nurse-manager's job to make patient rounds each morning, why not do so in the company of the team leader or primary nurse? During the rounds plans can be made for individualized nursing care and important messages can be communicated to assure that the plans will be implemented as they should. Through her first-hand observation of their work the nurse-manager can get some insight into the competence of her staff and perhaps find out about some of their learning needs and personal goals. What do they seem inept or confused about? What are they confident doing and where are they a little shaky? Perhaps during rounds she will find occasions to delegate tasks and to teach her staff some special aspects of patient care.

The point here is that if you want to have some control over your time, you must get that control by taking it. There really is no "free time" in your busy schedule unless you make it. Your time will be spent by others as long as you let them. If, however, you want to plan ahead, bring about change, and enjoy a sense of accomplishment in your work, it is up to you to set aside the time you need to reach your goals. An effective manager does not allow others to decide how her time will be spent. She sets her own priorities and makes decisions according to her personal values.

You also need to help those who work under you utilize their time efficiently. Try to view your work scene dispassionately and analytically. Exactly how are your employees spending their time? Is there a systematic use of work time or is everyone reacting to the pressures of the moment and then working slowly and aimlessly when the pressure is off? Do members of your staff concentrate on one activity (perhaps the one with the most visible results) and neglect others? What seem to be their priorities? What are your own? Do you know what you value most? Can you be flexible and change the routine so that time is used more effectively?

It might be helpful and informative for you and your employees to keep a kind of diary in which you record your daily work activities for one week. Specify the hour, the task performed, and the length of time spent performing each task. This need not be a minute-by-minute record, but it should be in enough detail to show a pattern of some kind. Later, as you review your week of work and see a pattern emerging you can detect certain behaviors that should be changed so that your time and that of your staff can be spent more constructively.

money

In your role of allocator of resources you must be aware of the budgetary and accounting systems of the institution in which you work. As a first-line manager you may not be concerned with planning a budget and deciding how funds will be distributed among the various departments and patient care units, but you are expected to work within the constraints of the budget that is in effect and do your share to control payroll costs and expenditures for equipment, supplies, and other items related to nursing services.

You should know what a budget is, the various kinds of budgets, their purposes, and your specific responsibilities in budgeting activities within the agency in which you work. The financial resources of any organization are actually spent, in large measure, by the employees who do the work. They are the ones who use the equipment and supplies. Employees who are wasteful in their use of supplies and abusive in their handling of equipment can undermine the best budgets. One of the major purposes of a budget is to control expenditures so that resources are evenly distributed among many different areas of need.

Tasks within the role of allocator of financial resources are not the same at different levels of management. It usually is the responsibility of high level executives to plan and implement *capital expenditure* budgets. These are related to long term goals involving changes in the physical plant—for example, replacement and renovation of old structures, expansion of facilities, and purchasing of major equipment. *Operating budgets* are usually prepared annually by each department within the agency. First-line managers may be expected to participate in planning operating budgets and to provide information at the time budgets are being revised.

An operating budget has two major components: The expense budget (the debit side of the ledger) and the revenue budget (the credit side). The budget for expenses projects such predetermined costs as salaries, equipment and supplies for a unit, and overhead. The budget for revenue predicts income from revenue-producing departments.[15] When projected expenses exceed projected revenue, decisions must be made on the basis of priorities of need. It is at this point that the first-line manager can provide valuable information so that decisions can be made fairly and objectively.

Your specific tasks in providing information for setting up and revising an operating budget might include your evaluation of disposable supplies to determine whether they are more or less economical than non-disposables. Because you are in a position to observe the use of equipment and evaluate first hand the products of different manufacturers you may be called upon to compare the products of different manufacturers and recommend those that prove to be the most economical in terms of dependability and durability. If you are responsible for requesting purchase of items needed on your unit, you should be specific and thorough in your evaluation. Your request should be submitted in writing. You must be able to validate the need for the item and provide information regarding manufacturer's name, length of warranty, expected time of delivery, and projected cost for installation (if any), and maintenance.[16]

Other tasks within the role of allocator of monetary resources might include devising and implementing a system of accountability for use of equipment and expenditure of supplies in your unit. Charges must be assigned to the bill of each patient and records kept and dispatched to the appropriate departments. If this is not done, the expense budget will undoubtedly exceed the revenue budget for your unit.

Taking inventory and systematically checking supplies are essential to effective budgeting. These tasks may be delegated by the nurse-manager to non-nursing personnel, but he/she must institute some check-points for control to avoid the extremes of empty shelves and frustrated workers and hoarded supplies and wastefulness.

people

Adequate coverage of a patient care unit with qualified personnel on duty 24 hours a day, seven days a week is a very real problem for nurse-managers at any level. Whether or not you are directly responsible for such coverage, you have some obligations in this area and should have competence in the performance of specific tasks within the role of allocator of personnel.

On a day-to-day or even an hour-to-hour basis, the first-line manager assigns nursing tasks to the nursing personnel working under her. These assignments should be made equitably and economically so that patients' nursing care needs are met and the overall patient care plan is implemented. Assignments are made according to informed choice; they are not left to chance. You do not use the "gozinta" method; that is, 3 (staff members) goes into 27 (patients) 9 times, therefore each staff member is assigned to care for 9 patients. An informed choice is one that is made only after determining each patient's nursing care needs during an 8-hour shift, and then selecting from available personnel the person or persons best suited to care for the patient.

You should be aware of various staffing patterns that might be employed to achieve the goal of adequate coverage. This means keeping abreast of current literature on staffing and being creative and innovative in your choice of patterns. One need not continue to staff a unit in a certain way just because that is how it has always been done. You should be a change agent when change is indicated.

The basic guideline in development of a method for staff utilization is that it be economical, stable, and equitable. Aside from the traditional concept of assigning individuals to specific tasks, there is a newer approach in which teams are scheduled to work in designated areas and are rotated to different shifts as a team. Other examples of innovative approaches to clinical staffing include the 10-hour day, 40-hour workweek, and a "premium day" to provide adequate coverage for weekends. The literature abounds with reports of staffing patterns that have been tried with varying degrees of success.

Participation in the agency's efforts to provide adequate coverage and quality patient care means taking part in studies to determine the kind of staff needed to meet the objectives of the agency. The studies are done to find answers to such questions as: How are staff members spending their time? What are they doing? Can some of the tasks performed by nursing personnel be delegated to non-nursing staff members?

The cost factors involved in obtaining quality health care continue to spiral upward. Consumers and third party payors such as private and governmental insurance agencies demand data to support requests for payment of the services of health care personnel. And, while it is ultimately the responsibility of nursing service administrators to compile and present the data, they cannot do this without the cooperation of first-line managers.

The general categories of the kinds of data needed have been identified by Warstler as:

- Factual information about the various types and degrees of nursing care needed by patients in a given hospital unit. The five levels of care needed are: intensive care, modified intensive care, intermediate care, minimal care, and self-care.

- Information found on the 24-hour general report that is prepared on each unit and submitted to the nursing service office before the end of each shift.

- Information that is helpful in determining total personnel hours required by patients in each of the above levels.[17]

Everyone in a managerial position in health care agencies shares responsibility for documenting the need for personnel. Despite protests about growing mountains of paper work, nurse-managers must face the realities of the old adage, "He who pays the piper calls the tune." We are in an age of accountability and that means written documentation and precise record keeping to justify the use of resources that are paid for by the consumer and taxpayer.

as handler of conflicts and grievances

In an environment as complex, varied, and changing as that found in most health-care organizations, conflicts and grievances are inevitable. Conflicts arises from unresolved differences of values, personalities, perceptions and expectations of role and unsuccessful communication and exchange of information. These differences and their resultant conflicts can be stimulating and occasions for growth. Conflict creates tension, but a certain amount of tension is healthy and conducive to a zestful and exciting life. Without conflict there is stagnation and death. The goal of the manager of conflict is to use the expected tensions of everyday living to advantage, as an impetus to change and an opportunity for growth.

Because conflict is so all-pervasive in the organizational setting, an entire chapter is devoted to the management of conflict. The tasks of the manager of conflict demand a high level of skill in interpersonal relationship and communication (see Chapter 9).

Grievances are defined as complaints that grow out of conflict. A person is aggrieved or dissatisfied because of circumstances that create discomfort. In the language of labor-management relations, a grievance is a formal complaint made under established grievance procedure. In collective bargaining between labor and management the grievance procedure clause is considered by labor leaders to be one of the most important clauses in the labor agreement.[18]

However, grievance procedures are not necessarily the outcome of union contracts. There are many non-union organizations that have grievance procedures for settling employee complaints. You should know the grievance procedure in the institution in which you work and follow it faithfully when the occasion arises. This means that you must develop your verbal and written communication skills. Try to maintain an open door to allow employees opportunity to air their grievances, and an open mind to receive their complaints without being judgmental. You should be able to write concise and factual statements, when called upon, to present management's point of view during a formal or informal grievance procedure. And there will be times when your subordinates will need your help in preparing their own cases when they feel they have a legitimate complaint against management. If this sounds as if you might be caught in the middle of a disagreement between labor and management, that is exactly what may happen. Your only recourse as first-line manager is to avoid taking sides and try to reserve judgment until the issue is clear. Then deal with the situation as honestly as you can.

Disciplinary cases comprise a large number of the grievances that are resolved by formal union-management procedures. Many of these time-consuming and sometimes emotionally traumatic negotiations could have been avoided if the first-line manager had been able to discipline employees fairly and communicate with them openly and honestly. Effective management of conflict requires an ability to appraise an employee's competence objectively and to support requests for reprimand, demotion, and dismissal with unbiased data. The handler of grievances should exercise self-discipline in order to avoid highly emotional and unfair confrontations with subordinates who have complaints about some aspect of their employment. Flexibility, a willingness to listen, and an ability to negotiate a settlement amicably are essential to effective management of conflict.

PERSONAL CHARACTERISTICS

We all have known nurse-managers who were paragons of efficiency, thoroughly competent in the performance of tasks within each managerial role, and yet who are lacking in that certain something that made working with them rewarding and enjoyable. Probably we also have had experience with less competent head nurses and supervisors who nevertheless have been the sort of person we would like to be when in charge of a patient unit. Somehow the personalities of these managers have compensated for whatever they lacked in knowledge and managerial skills. This is not to say that they were unable to carry out their responsibilities as they should, but rather that we held them in esteem, admired and respected them, and wanted to be like them. And, if they made a little mistake now and then, it was easy to forgive and forget.

In this section we will take a look at the attributes of an effective manager and try to be more specific in our description of desirable personality traits and behaviors of a person who is well suited for the job of manager. Admittedly, personality is less easily defined and measured than task performance, but it is worth examination for those who hope to become a manager that others would like to work with and emulate.

Teachers who manage classroom activities have a lot in common with nurse-managers. They work with others to set goals and objectives, subtly exert leadership, and serve as role models for those who work under their direction. In reporting research conducted to determine characteristics of "good vs. bad" teachers, Don Hamachek identified good teachers as those who (1) view teaching as primarily a human process involving human relations; (2) have a positive view of themselves, seeing themselves as basically and fundamentally "enough"; (3) have favorable opinions of others; (4) are well informed; and (5) are able to communicate what they know in a manner that makes sense to their students.[19]

If we were to take these characteristics and, substituting the word *managing* for *teaching*, and *subordinates* for *students,* we would have a workable description of the attributes of a good manager. As a further step in trying to analyze these characteristics, we might start to list behaviors that indicate how a person demonstrates these attributes as he/she functions in a managerial position.

The partially completed list of behaviors given below are those selected by participants in management classes and seminars. The behaviors listed in each category are not necessarily all that could be included, nor is a behavior listed under one heading necessarily excluded from the possibility of belonging in another. After reading the behaviors presented, you might want to observe someone you consider to be an effective manager and contribute your own findings.

- **Attribute:** *Views management as primarily a human process.*
    Behaviors:
    Asks subordinates to participate in setting objectives
    Has a sense of humor
    Smiles often
    Is kind but firm when disciplining others
    Praises staff when warranted
    Gives credit to staff members impartially
    Makes it possible for staff to attend meetings, classes, conferences.
    Is loyal to her staff members when she believes they have been
        wronged
    Tells the truth; does not "fudge" on facts
    Does not hold grudges

- **Attribute:** *Has a positive view of herself.*
    Behaviors:
    Admits her mistakes

Is willing to take risks

Counsels staff members who are not measuring up

Helps with patient care when needed

Clearly states her beliefs

Does what she considers right even if it is not the popular thing to do

Teaches staff members

Is well groomed

Accepts responsibility for her actions; does not try to put blame on others

Likes to see goals accomplished

Sees meaning in her work

- **Attribute:** *Has favorable opinions of others.*

  Behaviors:

  Delegates duties to others

  Listens to and acts on suggestions from subordinates

  Asks subordinates for help in solving problems

  Challenges staff members to suggest, plan, and implement change

  Allows staff members to accept responsibility for their own actions

  Does not ridicule subordinates who make a mistake

  Hears both sides of a story before making a judgment

  Ignores rumors; does not pass them along

  Encourages staff members to teach one another

  Encourages staff members to learn and try new techniques

- **Attribute:** *Is well informed.*

  Behaviors:

  Demonstrates knowledge of professional standards, goals, and issues

  Can speak knowledgeably about new techniques and tasks of nursing

  Keeps staff abreast of current techniques, etc.

  Attends in-service education and continuing education programs

  Reads nursing journals, management periodicals, and other professional literature

  Knows current policies, job descriptions, organizational charts and other aspects of organizational structure

- **Attribute:** *Is able to communicate what she knows in a manner that makes sense to subordinates.*

  Behaviors:

  Interprets goals and objectives of the agency to subordinates

  Explains treatments, diagnostic tests, procedures and policies in simple language

  Answers questions with short, to-the-point answers

  Asks questions one at a time

Explains what she is doing when demonstrating procedures to staff

Conducts short, well-planned staff conferences

Helps subordinates relate goals and objectives of agencies to their own personal goals.

As we have said, these personal characteristics and behaviors are those considered desirable from the perspective of nonmanagers. In spite of the fact that personal attributes and personality traits are not easily described, those who work under managers (and that includes most of us) can and do agree on the kind of things a good manager does or does not do in the work setting. Above all she refuses to compromise her principles and values for the sake of popularity. She challenges her staff members to grow and that means that sometimes they may be dissatisfied and not too happy with her or with themselves and their jobs. At other times they feel rewarded by a sense of accomplishment and pride in being a member of her team. In the words of Jay Hall, "Good managers challenge their people; poor ones comfort them."[20]

REFERENCES

[1]J. W. Hunt, *The Restless Organization*, (Sydney, Australia: John & Sons, Australasia Pty Ltd., 1972).

[2]F. E. Kast and J. E. Rosenzweig, *Organization and Management: A Systems Approach*, (New York: McGraw-Hill Book Co., 1970).

[3]J. Farley, "The climate for growth: The nurse's role in a changing hospital organization," *Supervisor Nurse*, (June, 1971), pp. 46-57.

[4]P. Drucker, *The Practice of Management*, (New York: Harper and Row, Inc., 1954).

[5]L. R. Sayles, *Managerial Behavior*, (New York: McGraw-Hill Book Co., 1964).

[6]J. W. Hunt, *op. cit.*, p. 32.

[7]H. Mintzberg, "The manager's job: Folklore and fact," *Harvard Business Review*, (July-Aug., 1975).

[8]M. R. Weisbord, "Why organizational development hasn't worked (so far) in medical centers," *Health Care Management Review*, (Spring, 1976).

[9]L. Jokenst, "Unit management: Separating myth from reality," *Hospital Progress*, (June, 1975).

[10]D. McGregor, "An uneasy look at performance appraisal," *Harvard Business Review*, (May-June, 1957).

[11]R. D. Gauerke, "Appraisal as a retention tool," *Supervisor Nurse*, (June, 1977).

[12]T. R. Tirney and N. Wright, "Minimizing the turnover problem: A behavioral approach," *Supervisor Nurse*, (Aug., 1973).

[13]H. Yura and M. Walsh, "Guidelines for evaluation: Who, what, when, where, and how," *Supervisor Nurse*, (Feb., 1972).

[14]T. F. Moore and E. Simendinger, "Evaluation as a two-way street," *Supervisor Nurse*, (June, 1976).

[14]A. Marriner, Budgets, *Supervisor Nurse*, (April, 1977).

[16]J. Froebe, "Scheduling: By team or individually," *Journal of Nursing Administration*, (May-June, 1974).

[17]M. E. Warstler, "Some management techniques for nursing service administrations," *Journal of Nursing Administration*, (Nov.-Dec., 1972).

[18]N. E. Amundson, "Grievance handling," *Journal of Nursing Administration*, (Sept.-Oct., 1972).

[19]D. Hamachek, "Characteristics of good teachers and implications for teacher education," *Phi Delta Kappan*, (Feb., 1969).

[20]J. Hall, "What makes a manager good, average, or bad?" *Psychology Today*, (Aug., 1976).

SUGGESTED READINGS

E. E. Beletz, "Some pointers for grievance handlers," *Supervisor Nurse*, (Aug., 1977).

T. M. Calender, "Improving working environment by improving administrative skills," *Supervisor Nurse*, (Sept., 1972).

M. R. Colton, "What is the manager's function in a health care facility?" *Supervisor Nurse*, (Sept., 1979).

J. Farley, "The climate for growth: The nurse's role in a changing hospital organization," *Supervisor Nurse*, (June, 1971).

N. D. Johnson, "The professional-bureaucratic conflict," *Journal of Nursing Administration*, (May-June, 1971).

S. A. LaRocco, "An introduction to role theory for nurses," *Supervisor Nurse*, (Dec., 1978).

B. N. Lawson, "Evaluation—A sorry procedure," *Supervisor Nurse*, (Oct., 1978).

M. L. McClure, "ANA standards for nursing services: Considerations in evaluation," *Supervisor Nurse*, (Aug., 1976).

E. N. Price, "Staffing: The most basic nursing service problem." *Supervisor Nurse*, (July, 1975).

I. G. Ramey, "Setting standards and evaluating care," *Journal of Nursing Administration*, (May-June, 1978).

E. B. Schwarz and R. A. MacKenzie, "Time-management strategy for women," *Journal of Nursing Administration*, (March, 1979).

chapter 3
index

chapter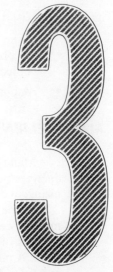
management as process
INTRODUCTION

In the previous chapter we analyzed the role of the manager and attempted to identify some of the functional and personality requirements for performance in the role. Another way in which the study of management might be approached is by analysis of the process, using as a framework the planning, organizing, and controlling functions of the manager.

In this chapter we will explore the notions that management is (1) problem-oriented, and (2) a systematic process that shares some of the same characteristics as the scientific method or research process and the nursing process; and that the problem-solving tasks of the manager follow a more or less sequential pattern according to the phases of the process.

These phases of problem-solving activities are given different names by various theorists, depending on the discipline in which each is working and the approach used to analyze the task of management. For purposes of organization and ease of presentation, the phases chosen and utilized in this chapter are:

- A *preprocess* of *discovery* phase in which the manager explores problem areas in the environment and tries to discover the kinds of problem that must be dealt with.

- A *data-gathering* phase that provides more clues and helps to identify a specific problem that needs immediate attention; the final activity in this phase is writing a clear and concise statement of the problem.

- A *planning* phase that involves setting goals and objectives for problem resolution.

- A phase of *implementing* the plans for achievement of goals and objectives.
- A phase of *evaluating* progress toward the goals.

MANAGEMENT IS PROBLEM-ORIENTED

Management is a problem-oriented process; the active manager analyzes problems and makes decisions throughout all the planning, organizing, and controlling functions of management.[1]

In the fields of medicine and nursing, the problem-oriented system of medical recordkeeping (POMR) provides a system for the methodical analysis of a patient's health needs and the planning of care to deal with them. A pioneer in this problem-oriented approach to the delivery of health care is Dr. Lawrence Weed, who first published his work in 1962.[2]

The problem-oriented approach to medical and nursing care and to management evolves from the traditional scientific method or research process. There are, therefore, parallel concepts and categories of functions related to the process of problem solving, regardless of the *environment* in which the problem develops, the *technological variables,* that is, the "things" used for dealing with the problem, and the individuals and groups of *people* who are working towards its resolution.

The parallels among the research process, the nursing process, and the management process have been noted by many theorists and authors. Essentially, the similarities are related to the steps or phases of the process. In research, or the scientific method, one first becomes aware of certain conditions or environmental elements that present problems, and attempts to identify or formulate a specific problem and state it in specific terms. This is followed by the collection of data through observation and, if possible, experiment. In the third phase the researcher formulates hypotheses or propositions that are tested or evaluated for confirmation.

Yura and Walsh describe four phases of the nursing process: assessing, planning, implementing, and evaluating.[3] The first phase involves gathering, analyzing, and interpreting data so that a problem or nursing diagnosis can be defined. This is followed by considering alternative actions, choosing one (decision-making) and developing a plan of action. The plan is then implemented through nursing activities, and in the final phase the results of these activities are evaluated to determine their effectiveness in accomplishing the objectives of the nursing care plan.

From your experiences in the use of the nursing process, you know that while the components of the process provide structure for the organization of nursing activities, you do not always proceed in an orderly, step-by-step manner, beginning with the first component and progressing through to the last. In response to input gathered in each phase you may look back to a previous component and change your diagnosis, plans or activities. For example, you might have established a nursing diagnosis on the basis of information gathered during assessment and chosen some nursing activities that you believed to be most effective in dealing with a patient's problem. Later, after having implemented these activities, you find that they are not working and a different approach must be taken and other nursing activities tried. The more knowledgeable, experienced, and skillful you become, the more easily you can manage the nursing process.

The phases of the management process are likewise concerned with assessment of the situation, gathering and analyzing data, identifying the problem, planning for its resolution, implementing the plan, and evaluating the outcome. Throughout the process the manager seeks feedback that might indicate a need to alter plans and activities so that the objective of problem resolution is more likely to be achieved.

THE SYSTEMATIC PROCESS OF MANAGEMENT

Process is defined by Webster as the action of moving forward progressively *on the way to* completion. A second definition states that process is the action of *continuously* going along through each of a succession of acts, events, and developmental stages.[4] From these definitions we can infer that process is chiefly concerned with the *behaving* or functional aspects of a system and its *becoming* or evolutionary aspects. These concepts were mentioned in Chapter 1 at the time when we discussed the definition and some very basic characteristics of a system. At that time it was noted that a system can be a human person, a group, a technological entity, or an organization.

One inference that might be drawn from the definition of process and the *becoming* nature of a system is that human beings are continuously in a state of realizing or actualizing their potential. People who are accomplishing their personal goals and developing their talents and abilities are self-actualizing, that is, they are in the process of becoming.

Maslow reminds us that we are all pilgrims on the way to a better life and that self-actualization is not a matter of achieving one great moment when a person is fully actualized. As he says, "It is not that on Thursday at four o'clock the trumpet blows and one steps into the pantheon forever and altogether. Self-actualization is a matter of degree, or little accessions accumulated one by one."[5]

If you accept the premise that human systems are in the process of becoming self-actualized, then it follows that organizations and their subsystems can also be self-actualizing in the sense that through the process of management, organizational and unit needs are being met and their objectives being achieved. It would be as unrealistic to look forward to the day that all of the problems on your patient care unit have been solved as it would be to look forward to the day that you and your subordinates have become completely self-actualized.

The definition of process does, however, imply that progress is being made. If you find yourself trying to resolve the same problem over and over again, you are not using the management process effectively. One of the hallmarks of successful first-line management is the resolution of *different* problems over a span of time. Another sign of progress is the achieving of your personal goals and those of your subordinates as well as those of the organizational system.

Systems, human or otherwise, are goal-oriented. Webster defines a system as *a complex unity formed of many often diverse parts subject to a common plan or purpose.* [6] An open system, such as a hospital, clinic, or one of their subsystems, is one that interacts with its environment. Because it is open, it allows for the necessary input-output transactions with the elements in its environment. Whatever is fed into a system, whether it is matter, energy, or information, is transformed in some way and then "put out" into the environment. For a system to remain viable it must have a feedback loop so that it can obtain information about how it is doing. This input guides the system in making the adjustments and adaptations necessary for its survival. (See Figure 3.1.)

When you are engaged in the process of management in an open system, the necessity for a feedback loop demands that you continually allow for two-way communication. The participative management approach permits communication in many directions, not merely the traditional one-way from-superior-to-subordinate route.

PHASES OF THE MANAGEMENT PROCESS

Traditionally nurses have been criticized for being "doers," the implication being that nurses don't spend much time sitting around thinking about things. The criticism is unfair, of course, but it arises from the fact that most nurses fully realize the necessity for getting on with it and getting the job done.

In 1966 Lois Knowles published a model for decision-making and problem-solving activities in nursing. In her model Knowles identified what she called the five "D's": discover, delve, decide, do, and discriminate. [7] These five components are similar to the five that we will use as a structural framework for describing what a first-line manager does when engaged in the process of management.

discovery

As explained earlier, this is a sort of preprocess phase that you have been involved in from the time you first began to reason. It is the preparatory stage during which you acquired and continue to accumulate

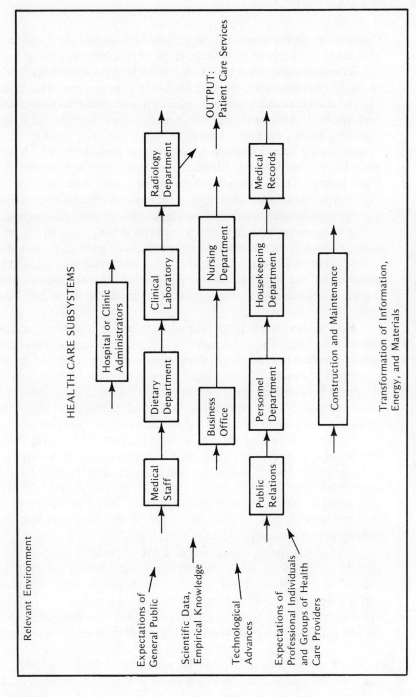

figure 3.1 subsystems of the health care system

HEALTH CARE SUBSYSTEMS

Relevant Environment

Expectations of General Public

Scientific Data, Empirical Knowledge

Technological Advances

Expectations of Professional Individuals and Groups of Health Care Providers

Hospital or Clinic Administrators

Medical Staff

Dietary Department

Clinical Laboratory

Radiology Department

Business Office

Nursing Department

Public Relations

Personnel Department

Housekeeping Department

Construction and Maintenance

OUTPUT: Patient Care Services

Transformation of Information, Energy, and Materials

the knowledge necessary to distinguish how things are from how they should be, and begin to classify the kinds of problems that you discover.

There are many ways by which you acquire the knowledge you need to recognize problems when they are present in your environment. Chaos, confusion, disorganization and wasted effort are recognizable wherever you find them. If you have had the experience of working in a smoothly operating patient care unit, you have had opportunity to learn how a subsystem should function when it is well managed. However, if you have never been in anything but a hectic, crisis-laden environment in nursing you might wonder if that is the way all patient care units function.

As you learn about, experience, and begin to practice effective management techniques you become more adept at discovering problems and identifying the general area in which a problem exists. There are four general areas in which problems in management might be located: (1) procedure, (2) policy, (3) interpersonal and intraorganizational relationships, and (4) lines of authority and span of control. Within each of these spheres of activity there are ever narrowing areas that lead eventually to the heart of the problem.

Here is an example of the use of knowledge, experience, and relevant information to facilitate discovery of the area in which a problem resides. At a conference for food service managers a participant stated that she had a problem of communication with nurses. As a matter of fact, many, if not all, problems in management can be called "communication problems", so there was a need to get more information and be more specific. As the participant continued to describe the situation it was learned that she was responsible for preparing food to be served to patients in a long term health care facility. Some patients ate in the dining room when they were feeling up to leaving their rooms and others had trays brought to their bedside. The trouble was that the food service operator "never" knew which patients were going to the dining room and which were eating in their rooms. It was very difficult for her to plan from day to day and have the necessary number of trays prepared ahead of time.

Further discussion revealed that a list of patients needing trays to be served in their rooms was compiled every night during the 11-7 shift and sent to the diet kitchen every morning. So there was some communication taking place. The list was completed by nursing personnel on each unit, but in the words of the food service manager, "They take their time getting it to me and usually sit around talking to one another before they bother to send it."

Now we begin to see that we have a different kind of problem. Not so much one of communication (a list *was* compiled and sent each day) as one of interpersonal relationships and an understanding of the duties of nurses in regard to giving morning report at the change of shifts. It also requires some awareness on the part of the nursing staff that food service personnel start planning for breakfast long before 7:30 a.m. It is doubtful that sending a memo to the nurses to get the list in on time would be as effective as a plan to have personnel from the two departments share their concerns and come to an agreement about how the problem could be resolved. The breakdown in communication was the result, not the cause of the trouble. When interpersonal relationships are involved, resolution of the problem of politics will improve communication, not the other way round.

Like all other phases of the management process, discovery is continuous and ongoing. As new knowledge about sound management practice is acquired, awareness is heightened and discovery made easier. The other phases also contribute to this awareness because the components are interrelated and not as clearly delineated as they might appear to be.

data gathering and analysis

This phase, comparable to the assessment phase of the nursing process, has as its objective the identification of a problem. It involves data gathering, analysis of the information received, and preparing a written statement of the problem. Having gone through the discovery phase you are aware that a problem does exist. Your goal now is to find out precisely what the problem is.

There are many kinds and sources of data that will help with identification of a management problem. Authorities suggest that you gather as much data as possible, even more than probably you will need. At some point you must decide which data are relevant and which are not. The most successful problem solvers are those who can distinguish between information that helps define the problem and that which only muddies the waters.

Not only must the data be *relevant,* but the sources of information must be *reliable.* Reliability refers to consistency, and so the facts being received should not be in conflict with one another. If for example, there seems to be a problem with keeping accurate records of intake and output, there should be evidence from a number of sources, all of it consistently pointing to the conclusion that the recording of intake and output leaves something to be desired. Such sources might include physicians' complaints, the patients' charts, absence of any visible means by which intake and output information is being obtained and recorded throughout the eight-hour shift, statements by staff members that the procedure is or is not being done as it should, and so on. Remember that this phase involves obtaining and compiling factual information. If there is sufficient evidence that the records are inadequate and inaccurate, then the data are relevant and reliable.

Keeping the incoming data relevant, rejecting information that is not significant to the problem, and determining whether the evidence is from a reliable source is not easy. One must keep a cool head and persist in concentrating on the issue at hand. Problems in management usually arouse emotions in the persons involved, especially when there is some inference that somebody is not doing his/her job well. People become defensive and use all sorts of mechanisms for refusing to face up to the problem and diverting attention away from it.

There are some things the nurse-manager can do to help avoid an accusatory atmosphere and defensiveness in herself as well as in members of her staff. Concentrate on the task or function that is being done poorly or not at all. Never mind, at this point at least, trying to find out who is to blame or what is the basic cause of the problem. Your objective is to collect evidence that will be helpful in pinpointing the problem. You do not blame a patient for becoming dehydrated. You gather data for assessment and then decide whether or not the problem of dehydration does indeed exist. You do not allow yourself to be distracted from identifying problems of management by looking for its cause or contemplating possible solutions. That comes later. During this second phase of the process you are concerned with gathering information that will help you determine exactly what the problem is.

You must set priorities in choosing management problems that need immediate attention just as you must for nursing problems. If you have gathered more information than you really need for one problem, which you are well advised to do, then you are going to find that there are quite a few problems.

The multiplicity of problems is to be expected when you are working in a complex and dynamic system. You are not going to resolve them all at once. Remember that progress is made in short steps, beginning with the handling of those problems that you decide are most crucial and most likely to interfere with your goal of a high level of patient care.

writing a problem statement

After having gathered and analyzed data pertinent to the problem, it is necessary to *write a statement of the problem* as you see it. There are very good reasons for having a written statement. If it is not written down you will have great difficulty refining it. The more specific you are in stating the problem the more likely you are to find a workable solution.

The evolution of a problem statement might be seen in the following:

First draft: *Staff is spending too much time during morning report at the change of shifts.* Questions not answered: Which staff members? All or some? Those who are coming on duty or those going off? Do night shift personnel fail to give report correctly or are day shift personnel unavailable, late, or already starting their own day's work? Are they inattentive? Interruptive? Is there a system by which some staff members who are coming on duty will answer call lights while nighttime personnel give reports? What is happening during change of shifts? What are nursing attendants, team leaders, charge nurse, ward secretary, and others doing while report is being given?

Second draft: *Charge nurse for night shift is not able to give a concise and comprehensive report.* After observing her during report and talking with her, you find that she needs help in preparing for report and deciding what is pertinent and what need not be reported.

Third draft: *Charge nurse for night shift needs instruction in the correct way to give report at the change of shifts.* Now you have a problem statement that points to a relatively easy solution. You are ready to move to the next phase of the management process — planning for achievement of objectives that will lead to resolution of the problem.

As you may have noticed, it is likely that in the gathering of additional information to refine your written statement, other problems could be identified. Perhaps there should be a more orderly system for carrying on the business of the day while report is given. For example, who should be answering call lights, communicating with physicians, visitors, personnel from other departments who are on the unit, answering the phone, and so on? Perhaps one or two members of the staff receiving report need to be counseled about their rude behavior during report.

Writing a definition of the problem is more than just writing a statement. It is itself a process of systematic delving for information, analysis of data, and interpretation of data to reach valid conclusions about what is really going on. Just as the whole management process is cyclic in nature, so, too, is each component. Once the problem or problems have been identified you are well on your way toward planning for their resolution.

planning

During this phase you will be making decisions about your goal for resolution of the problem that has been identified and the objectives that will lead to accomplishment of the goal. The goal and objectives constitute an orderly plan for progress.

The manner in which the decisions are made and the plan devised will depend on your choice of leadership style. Remember that contingency management means choosing the style and techniques that suit the situation. It is up to you to decide whether or not you will involve subordinates in the decision making and planning, and the extent to which they will be involved. If you choose to make the decisions and then sell your subordinates on your ideas and plans, you must be prepared to communicate frequently with the persons who will be affected by your decisions.

The *goal* for resolution of the problem gives meaning and purpose to the plan of action. It must be clearly stated from the outset so that it can serve as a guide for developing measurable objectives. During this phase of the management process you will be answering the question, "What can be done about the problem?'' Your goal must be realistic or it is doomed to failure. You should consider all resources available and the potential of each one for helping reach the objectives.

When deciding what will be done, who will do it, how it is to be done, when, where, and at what cost, you are going to have to draw upon a large deposit of skills and knowledge. Not only are you limited by the constraints of time, people, and money, you also must take into account your own strengths and weaknesses. In other words, don't be unrealistic about the things you can reasonably expect to do and your willingness to expend the necessary time and energy.

It is not a reflection on you as a person to honestly admit that at this stage of your development you have not had the experience and training needed to be fully competent in all areas of nurse-management. With self-analysis comes self-acceptance. You are a self-actualizing person in the process of becoming self-actualized.

Taking as an example the problem statement that was developed during the second phase, you should consider whether you or someone else is better qualified to instruct the 11-7 charge nurse. How competent is she in learning on her own if you provide her with reading material on the topic? Do you know what learning materials are available to you and to her? How will you approach her to inform her of the need to improve? Will you decide what she needs to know or are you willing to spend time talking with her to help identify her own learning needs?

knowledge, skills and attitudes

The more *knowledge* a person has at hand when making a decision, the more valid that decision will be. When deciding on the goal for resolution of the problem it would be helpful to know:

- How others have effectively resolved similar problems.
- What is considered to be the ideal in the areas of procedure, policy, organizational structure, and interpersonal relationships.
- What is realistic in terms of resources available for reaching the ideal.

During this phase the *skills* needed include an ability to write objectives that are measurable and easily understood. There is little point in setting up objectives if you have no way of knowing whether or not they are ever accomplished. You also will need skills in written and verbal communication so that everyone involved fully understands the plan of action. If the planned activities extend over a period of time, you will need to set up objectives that allow for periodic checkpoints for control. At these checkpoints you might make provision for feedback from the staff in order to determine whether changes in the objectives should be made to make the plan more workable.

Finally, there will be a need for *attitudes* of confidence in yourself and your staff. You should be convinced that the plan is workable and that all of you are capable of making it work. You should be flexible so that if change is necessary you will be able to accept the necessary revisions. It really isn't much fun to have to face up to the fact that your plans were not all perfect from the beginning, but it certainly is easier to accept if you recognize from the outset that changes probably will be made. Above all, you should feel that making decisions and planning for improvement are challenging and worthwhile.

implementing

It is apparent from the title of the phase that this is the time during which the decisions you have made and the planning that has been done will be put into action. Here is where you will bring to bear all that you know and all the skills you have developed in motivation, delegation, and communication. You probably will find also that during this phase you are learning more about yourself and your staff.

Don't be surprised if implementation of the plan uncovers several other problems that need attention. Just don't let them distract you from your goal unless, of course, they present insurmountable obstacles. If one or more problems simply must be dealt with before you can make any progress, then you must postpone, *not necessarily discard,* your plan and return to phase two. You may not have realized it, but you were going through phase one when you began to discover new problems while trying to deal with your original one.

Returning to phase two, you identify the problem that is so troublesome, give it top priority and decide how it can be resolved. This is an example of the cyclic nature of the management process. It is *not* an indication that you are not utilizing the management process correctly. On the contrary, it may very well indicate that you understand the concept and are experiencing it in the real world of management.

During the phase in which you put your plan into action you may have occasion to use several different styles of leadership. These are discussed later in this text. At this point we will simply point out that leadership skills are essential to successful implementation of the plan. When checking the progress of the plan you should be able to communicate your findings so that staff members know whether or not they are doing what is expected of them. They, in turn, should have opportunities to share their evaluation of the feasibility of the plan.

Attitudes that are important to successful completion of this phase include a willingness to persist when others become discouraged. If there is evidence that what is being done is effective, even though it may entail hard work and perseverance, you should be able to maintain your own enthusiasm and transfer that enthusiasm to your staff. If, however, the plan proves to be too ambitious and not workable in its present form, you may have to stop and revise it so that it is more realistic.

multiplicity and complexity

Sometimes you might wonder whether the management process can be of any value in resolving what appears to be a monumental problem of management. A problem that appears to be overwhelming could, on analysis, prove to be a conglomerate of smaller problems that can be resolved or at least alleviated when dealt with one at a time.

In contrast, complex problems are those that are fuzzy, pervasive, hard to delineate, and qualitative rather than quantitative. Complex problems do not lend themselves to resolution by a scientific and methodical process. To attempt resolution of problems that are related to values and attitudes with the expectation that there is one right answer to be found is to set yourself up for disappointment and disillusionment. On the other hand, to consider every problem beyond your capabilities is to admit that you cannot function effectively as a manager. Let's use the following incident as an example of the management process at work.

Mrs. Dove is a team leader for a nursing care team composed of one LPN and two nursing attendants. She defined her problem as follows: *I do not feel confident that my team members are always able to carry out their assignments during the day.*

Mrs. Dove consulted with her team members and enlisted their help in planning and implementing a solution to the problem. They agreed to a goal of periodic meetings during the eight-hour shift for the purpose of apprising the leader of difficulties they might be having or to assure her that things were going well for them. They devised a plan whereby the team leader would meet each team member at the nurses' station every hour and give a brief report of their progress in completing assignments up to that point. If one member was not able to keep up with her scheduled activities, one of the others would volunteer to help out until she caught up. If either the team leader or a team member could not be available at the designated time, she would leave a note on the bulletin board saying where she could be reached.

After three days it became apparent that hourly meetings were impossible because they were interrupting patient care and took too much time. The plan was revised so that meetings took place every two hours unless there was something urgent that needed to be communicated to the team leader. In that case the team member involved was to find the leader and inform her of the difficulty.

The new plan worked fairly well and met with minimal resistance from the team members because they came to realize that meeting with the team leader actually took less than a few minutes and had the advantage of getting the help they needed to complete their assignments. The team leader discovered that she was better prepared to give a report at the end of the shift because she had a good idea of what had happened during the day. The plan gave the team leader the reassurance she was seeking. The members developed a sense of belonging to a group that was working together to accomplish mutual goals.

During implementation and revision of the plan the team leader became aware of a need for one of the members to improve her competence and speed in the performance of several nursing procedures. Identification of this newly discovered problem led the team leader into the management process cycle again.

evaluating

Evaluation is the measurement of an event, characteristic, behavior, or other subject against predetermined criteria. Criteria are standards by which one makes a judgment about the quality or worth of something. In the evaluating phase of the management process the outcome criteria are determined by the goal and objectives of the plan. An objective is what is hoped to be accomplished in the future. Outcome criteria state what should have been accomplished as a result of certain activities.

Evaluation occurs throughout all phases of the management process, influencing and being influenced by the activities in each phase. The example of Mrs. Dove and her team members shows how ongoing evaluation prompted them to revise their plan. However, the final phase of evaluation should be centered on how well objectives and goals have been met.

The content of the objectives identified during the deciding phase help determine who will conduct the evaluation and how it is to be done. If the objectives centered on one person, as in the case of the charge nurse on the night shift needing to improve her competence in giving report, then the evaluation focuses on her. She should, therefore, take part in the final phase of discrimination. The nurse-manager who worked with her to improve her ability to give report at the change of shifts also should participate in this evaluation. Together they decide whether the objectives that they set forth were reached.

There will be times when group decisions are made and plans drawn up and implemented by a group. In these instances the group looks at their objectives, translates them into outcome criteria, and measures results of the plan against these criteria.

Taking the objectives of Mrs. Dove and her team members to illustrate how objectives are converted into outcome criteria, we could write the following:

- *Goal:* Reassurance of team leader will be accomplished by periodic communication with and direction of team members.
- *Objectives:*

    Who: Team leader and *all* team members.

    What: Will meet to report progress and receive directions as needed.

When: At 9:00, 11:00 a.m. and 1:00 p.m. every day.

Where: Nurses' station.

At what cost: No more than five minutes of the leader's time at each session, less for each team member.

- *Outcome Criteria*

    1. Team leader and each of her members met daily at 9:00, 11:00, and 1:00 at the nurses' station.

    2. Team members and leader left message on bulletin board when they were unable to be at the nurses' station at designated times.

    3. Questions were asked and answered, information freely exchanged in regard to completion of assignments.

    4. Team members needing additional help and advice received them when needed.

    5. Team leader became more confident that each team member was completing her assignments on schedule.

Any observer, even an outsider who did not know the whole story about identification of the problem, revision of the plan, and formulation of objectives could use these criteria and make a valid distinction between the criteria that were met and those that were not.

Let us emphasize again how important it is that goals, objectives, and criteria be put into writing. When one is working in a busy and distracting environment, it is easy to forget details. But these are the elements that can enhance or impede progress through the process. Having details in writing serves as a guide for all who are expected to work toward reaching the goal. One of the most important competencies of a successful manager is the ability to attend to detail.

Criteria are standards based on knowledge or assumptions about how things should be. These standards are derived from job descriptions, personnel policies, departmental objectives, standards of nursing practice, and written procedures. The nurse-manager and all of her subordinates should have ready access to the standards pertinent to the fulfillment of their specific tasks. They should be knowledgeable about the standards and their implications for the practice of nursing at all levels. The appraisal of employee competence is covered more fully in Chapter 10.

We have said that definitions of management usually include the words *planning, directing,* and *controlling* because they are considered to be the essential functions of management. As you look over the phases of the management process you can see that the five phases of the process describe more precisely how one goes about carrying out these basic functions.

Although the management process is problem oriented, that is not to say that utilizing the components of the process will always lead to resolution of a problem. In the event that the process does not produce resolution, you have three alternatives: (1) You can try a different strategy for resolution; (2) you can go back and reformulate the problem; or (3) you can give up trying to resolve a particular problem.

To accept the fact that a problem cannot be completely resolved is not necessarily an admission of defeat unless, of course, you allow yourself to get into a win-lose situation with no room for compromise and reconciliation. As long as there is a balance of power and you can maintain some sense of control, some problems can be managed so that they do not create unbearable tension and stress, even though they are not completely resolved. If, however, a problem creates an intolerable working environment in which no compromise is acceptable to you, the only recourse is to seek employment elsewhere. If the problem does not create unbearable circumstances, it may be best to ignore it. Not all problems *can* be or necessarily *must* be resolved.

REFERENCES

[1]R. A. MacKenzie, "The management process in 3D," *Harvard Business Review,* (Nov.-Dec., 1969).

[2]L. L. Weed, *Medical Records, Medical Education, and Patient Care,* (Cleveland: Press of Case Western Reserve University, 1971).

[3]H. Yura and M. B. Walsh, *The Nursing Process,* 3rd ed., (New York: Appleton-Century-Crofts, 1978).

[4]*Webster's Third New International Dictionary,* (Chicago: G.&C. Merriam Co., 1971).

[5]A. H. Maslow, *The Farther Reaches of Human Nature,* (New York: The Viking Press, 1971).

[6]Webster, *op. cit.*

[7]L. N. Knowles, "Decision-making in nursing and necessity for doing," *ANA Clinical Sessions, 1966,* (New York: Appleton-Century-Crofts, 1967).

SUGGESTED READINGS

R. Chin, "The utility of system models and developmental models for practitioners," *Nursing Digest,* Vol. VI, No. 4, (Winter, 1979).

P. Menkin, "How a group can help solve your problems," *Nursing 75.* (July, 1975).

M. A. Rossworm, "A human resource framework for administrative practice," *Supervisor Nurse,* (Aug., 1978).

R. C. Swanwberg, "Planning—a function of nursing administration, Part I and Part II," *Supervisor Nurse,* (April, 1978 and May, 1978).

R. Veninga, "Interpersonal feedback: a cost-benefit analysis," *Journal of Nursing Administration,* (Feb., 1975).

P. Wong, et al., "Problem solving through process management," *Journal of Nursing Administration,* (Jan., 1975).

chapter 4
index

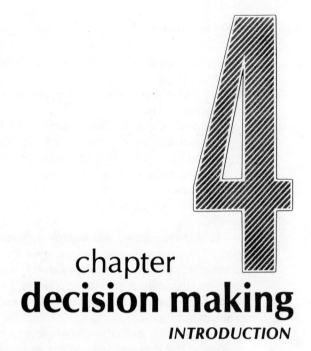

chapter
decision making

INTRODUCTION

Decision making is one of the major tasks of problem solving. In Chapter 3 we described management as a problem-solving process with components similar to those of the nursing process. In each of the components described in Chapter 3, decisions are made and alternative courses of action are chosen at critical points. The consequences of each of these decisions have some impact on the outcome or end results of the problem-solving process.

Managers engage in decision making, whether consciously or unconsciously, throughout every day of their lives, as, in fact, we all do as long as we are alive and aware of and able to respond to whatever is going on around us. By virtue of their positions in the organizational hierarchy, managers have the authority to make certain kinds of decisions and the concomittant responsibility for their consequences. Thus the careers of managers at all levels are either favorably or adversely affected by the decisions they make.

The decisions made by first-line managers may not involve expenditures of large amounts of money or other resources of the organization, but the kinds of decisions that they do make, or refuse to make because of lack of initiative, are no less important to the health and survival of the organization. Evaluations of the competence and effectiveness of a first-line manager are based in large measure on the quality of the decisions he/she makes and his/her willingness to accept the risks and responsibilities of a decisive leader.

Decision theorists are interested in providing guidelines so that the element of risk is reduced and the outcome is more predictable. Mathematicians and computer scientists can structure a response so that there is a very high level of certainty about the consequences of a decision and therefore a greatly reduced level of risk. But not all decisions lend themselves to programmed responses. Those that involve human interaction, values, attitudes, and behaviors are and probably always will be subject to some uncertainty and risk.

Through the years researchers from many disciplines have focused their attention on the kinds of decisions made by managers, the characteristics and behavior of successful decision makers, and the criteria by which a decision might be objectively evaluated. The three levels at which decision making has been and continues to be studied are: (1) the decision-making process, (2) the decision maker(s), and (3) the decision itself.[1]

In this chapter we will discuss decision making at each of these three levels. The process is a series of mental and physical activities in which the decision maker becomes aware of the need to make a decision, identifies the problem, compiles a list of alternative paths toward its resolution, and selects from these alternatives one that appears to be most likely to lead to problem resolution.

The decision maker might use one or more approaches to the task of deciding. These range from the totally rational and computational approach of the computer, to the totally unprogrammable approach, as in the resolution of "one of a kind" problems for which there is no known precedent on which to make a judgment. We will discuss this continuum of decision making and suggest some guidelines and techniques used in various approaches.

Evaluation of the decision itself might be viewed from the perspective of the decision maker and from that of the administration of the organization in which he/she is employed. We will identify some of the criteria by which a decision could be evaluated.

THE DECISION-MAKING PROCESS

Some of the earliest studies of decision making viewed the process as a rational and logical progression toward predictable outcomes. Purely rational decision making requires that the decision maker: (1) know all the variables in the situation; (2) know all the alternatives available; and (3) be able to choose the one alternative that will meet all the objectives of the decision maker.

In reality, managers cannot possibly know all the variables in a situation as complex as those encountered in the work setting, nor can they prepare an all-inclusive list of alternatives. As a sort of compromise, a "quasi-rational" approach is used so that the consequences of a decision can be expected in terms of *probabilities* rather than *certainties*. Such an approach gives the decision maker some control over what is happening when dealing with complex problems, but it does not necessarily guarantee that the desired outcomes will be achieved.

For example, you might logically assume that if you decide to delegate some responsibility for the orientation of new personnel to one of your subordinates, then you will have more time to devote to tasks that cannot be delegated. Your decision is a rational one to the extent that you have considered as many of the variables in the situation as you can, given the constraints of time, limited knowledge, and other conditions. Some of the more important considerations would be the willingness and ability of the subordinate to accept the responsibility, your own level of competence in delegating, and the expected reaction of the new staff members. After taking these variables into account, you can predict that your objective of having more time *probably* will or will not be reached, but you cannot say that it *certainly* will or will not be.

Researchers in rational decision making as it has just been described are concerned with the three basic questions proposed by John Dewey in the early nineteen hundreds. These questions are: (1) What is the problem? (2) What are the alternatives? (3) Which alternative is best?[2]

Using the work of Dewey as a starting point, Katz and Kahn attempted to identify some of the factors that influence the decision-making process. Their goal was to provide some structure to the activities of decision-making so that guidelines could be developed and decisions could be made more rationally.[3] They did not intend the components of the process to be a fool-proof recipe for making decisions and resolving problems. A step-by-step methodology is not compatible with the concept of process as a dynamic phenomenon.

The four stages of the decision-making process proposed by Katz and Kahn are: (1) pressures from the environment that create a feeling of stress in the person or persons who are the decision makers; (2) analysis of the type of problem at hand and its definition or dimensions; (3) search for alternatives; and (4) consideration of the consequences of each alternative solution and making a final choice from among them.

awareness of the problem

Decision-making starts when a person or persons begin to feel uncomfortable about what they perceive to be a discrepancy between how things actually are and how they believe they should be. At this point it is not clear to them exactly what the problem is. They may be unable even to give a rational explanation for their feelings of stress and tension, but they believe that a decision of some kind is called for.

If the problem-causing disequilibrium and discomfort are important to the individual or group, there is an attempt to deal with it in some way. These attempts will require some decision making, rational or otherwise, to find relief. Some individuals who encounter problems at work might choose to avoid the problem by removing themselves from the situation—physically, by quitting their jobs or requesting a transfer, or psychologically, by remaining aloof and using some mental escape mechanisms such as rationalizing. Others will confront the issue and seek ways to resolve the problem in some fashion. The thoughts and actions that follow the initial decision to do something about a troublesome situation are the remaining components of the process.

identifying the problem

This is perhaps the most difficult phase of the process and one that frequently is glossed over rather quickly as the decision maker anxiously moves on to the tasks of searching for and selecting alternatives. It is unfortunate that we have this tendency to get on with resolving a problem before we are sure exactly what it is that needs resolving. It is rather obvious that if a problem is not identified accurately and its cause diagnosed correctly, there is a good possibility that an appropriate and rational alternative for its resolution will not be found. And yet it is not uncommon for people who think of themselves as having a good share of common sense to begin considering alternatives before they have analyzed the problem and gotten down to the basic issue.

When you start to analyze a problem, remember that your goal is to make an explicit statement about the nature of the problem and its probable cause. At this point try to resist the temptation to search for alternatives; discipline yourself to get to the heart of the problem first. This is not easy to do, but it gets less difficult with experience.

In Chapter 3 we talked about the discovery phase of problem solving and the general areas in which a management problem might be located. These areas were related to structural elements of the organization, such as procedure, policies, chain of command, and areas of responsibility; and interpersonal relationships and conflicts between individuals and groups within the organization. When you are trying to answer the question, **"What is the problem?", you might ask yourself such questions as: Is it related to structure? What aspect of structure is involved? Is it a matter of** ignorance of rules and regulations or one of ignoring them? Is there a clash of personalities, values, objectives? Are personal objectives of one or more staff members incompatible with the objectives of the patient care unit?

Identifying problems requires skill in analysis of the situation and asking the right kinds of questions. Some people are more adept at analyzing than others, but we all can improve our analytic skills by looking for relationships among the various elements of a situation. We draw from a store of past experience and knowledge of similar situations and from our perception of what is right and proper.

If you are comfortable with a participative style of leadership, the knowledge and experiences of your subordinates can make a significant contribution to the store of knowledge. (Methods of decision making for groups are discussed later in this chapter.) The more sources of information you have, the larger the body of information you can draw from. It is important that you get as many facts as you possibly can before identifying the problem or making a diagnosis. When you are trying to identify a management problem, be sure that you talk with all of the people involved.

To illustrate, some of your subordinates have complained about the behavior of the relief charge nurse, who comes from an adjacent patient care unit to work in your place on your days off. They are unhappy because they do not know what she expects of them. She divides the work load differently, uses a different system for developing nursing care plans on newly-admitted patients, and becomes upset when they do not carry out assignments as she wants them done. They suspect that she wants the job of head nurse on your unit and that is why she makes changes that she thinks of as improvements.

At first glance it does seem possible that the problem is one of interpersonal conflict between the relief nurse and your subordinates. However, after consultation with her alone and then with her *and* your subordinates, it is determined that she is not aware that she is doing things differently. She has not observed you at work, nor has she had adequate orientation to your unit and the way you do things. The subordinates complain that they do not know what she expects of them, but she does not know what you and they expect of her.

Once you are reasonably sure that you have identified the problem and found its probable cause, you are ready to consider some alternatives and select the one that appears most likely to either minimize the effects of the problem or resolve it completely. As you can see from the above example, it would have been very easy to have considered the problem to be one of jealousy, ambition, or a critical attitude on the part of the relief head nurse. Any alternative action aimed at resolving interpersonal problems by confronting her with her apparent criticism of the way you run your unit probably would have created even more problems.

search for information and alternatives

During this phase the decision maker gathers facts and data from a variety of sources, including his/her own past experiences and observations. Information is said to be the raw material of the decision-making process. It is gathered from the external and internal environments of the decision maker, sifted and weighed, judged relevant or irrelevant to the problem at hand, and transformed into action-oriented alternatives for problem resolution.

In your search for information you might use both formal and informal networks or channels of information. Much of the information you receive will be verbally transmitted through conversations with your subordinates, colleagues, friends, and superiors. On a rather informal basis you might ask how they perceive the problem, what they see as possible alternatives for its resolution, and what other sources of information, verbal or written they might suggest. These sources could be within the structure of organization, as for example, written policies, procedures, and *standing plans*, or they could include professional journals, textbooks, and other printed materials obtained from outside sources.

Standing plans are of interest to you because they are made available to managers who must deal with *recurrent and routine* problems that can be handled with dispatch. Such plans limit the alternatives available to the manager; one can either follow the plan or choose to be more creative, but along that path may lie disaster for a first-line manager. An example of a standing plan is the grievance procedure that organizations usually have prepared in advance so that problems related to formal complaints by employees can be handled objectively and consistently. The first-line manager is expected to follow standing plans unless otherwise directed.

Problems that are unique require a more extensive search for information. Most formal channels of communication in an organization are fairly well defined. Memos about policy and procedure are passed along specified routes, and staff meetings are held to bring managers and subordinates up to date and keep them current with the structural elements of the organization.

Informal channels of information are typified by the grapevine. Never underestimate the effectiveness of the grapevine for sending and receiving information quickly, efficiently, and—you may be surprised to learn—accurately. Studies of grapevines in organizations have shown that they are 80 to 95 percent accurate in the information that is passed along.

In accumulating and processing information, you will be concerned with accuracy, but you also must be sure that the information is relevant to the problem and useful in helping you develop a list of alternatives. A problem that has been identified as one of incompetence on the part of one of your subordinates will require information that is different from that needed to resolve a problem of absenteeism.

The search for information and the listing of alternatives continues until the decision maker finds as many alternatives as he/she thinks are needed to make the final choice. The number of alternatives generated will depend on the approach or mode chosen by the decision maker. If the *satisficing or satisfying* mode is used, the search will end as soon as the decision maker finds an alternative that he/she thinks will meet most of the needs and objectives that have been identified. A *maximizing or optimizing mode* is one in which the decision maker continues to search for information and alternatives until the best approach at least cost is found. Later on, when we discuss the decision maker, we will see that personality, values, and other factors influence the mode that is utilized.

making a choice

The better informed you are, the better prepared you will be to develop a list of feasible alternatives and select from it an alternative that you believe to be the best under the circumstances. In making the selection you will consider the anticipated consequences of your decision. For example, you will need to ask yourself how well the decision will be accepted by others. Decisions usually bring about change, and with change comes the possibility of conflict. Acceptance of a decision and the adjustments it will require, either in values or task performance or both, must always be taken into consideration. If people must implement your decision, then you need to identify those people and know what kinds of adjustments you will be asking them to make.

The process of decision making is concerned with achieving objectives and goals; that is, closing the gap between existing conditions and the perceived ideal, and removing obstacles to the attainment of goals. In the selection of alternatives you will need to consider the number and kind of objectives that you hope to accomplish by your decision. You must be realistic about the resources needed to carry out the decision and how they compare with the personnel, time, money and material that are accessible. Additionally, you need to restrict the number of objectives to a manageable size. Bear in mind that self-actualization of individuals and organizations means progress in small increments. Your chances of success in implementing and sustaining a decision are better if you keep your objectives within reasonable limits.

Let's say, for example, that your subordinates have demonstrated an unwillingness to deal with parents who stay with their children on your pediatric unit. One of the goals of the unit is to enlist and encourage co-operation of the parents in the care of their children during hospitalization. Many of your staff members frustrate accomplishment of this goal by either ignoring the parents or discouraging them from doing anything for their children. In order to move closer to the attainment of your goal of cooperation between nurses and parents you will need to develop some realistic short-term objectives. Some of the more critical of these might be:

* Review of goals of the unit with subordinates.
* Opportunities for subordinates to express their feelings about the goal in question and whether they think it is a good idea to let parents participate in the care of hospitalized children.

- Help from the in-service education staff in setting up unit conferences focusing on the rationale for, and helpful techniques in working with, the parents.
- Leaders for the conferences from among the subordinates who are least resistant to the notion of participative care.

A list of objectives might be written in chronological order; that is, you identify the one that needs to be done first, then second, and so forth through a logical sequence. The objectives also should be ranked in order of importance so that in the event time becomes a crucial factor, you can select those that are most important and omit those that are not so critical to implementation of your decision.

THE DECISION MAKER

On a decision-making continuum the range extends from decisions that are totally programmable to those that are nonprogrammable.[4] (See Figure 4.1.) A decision maker can be a person, a group, or in this age of computer technology, a machine. Totally programmed decisions can be made by a computer and the outcome predicted with mathematic certainty. Other decisions that are near the programmed end of the continuum are those made according to standing plans developed to deal with routine problems. The standing orders written by physicians and the routines for preparing patients for diagnostic tests are examples of programmed decisions for the management of patient care. Grievance procedures for handling formal complaints by employees have already been mentioned as examples of standing plans.

Routine or programmed situations have relatively predictable outcomes. The decision maker already has a set of responses to the stimulus for making a decision. In the organization in which you work there probably are policies and procedures to guide you in making decisions in a number of

figure 4.1   decision-making continuum

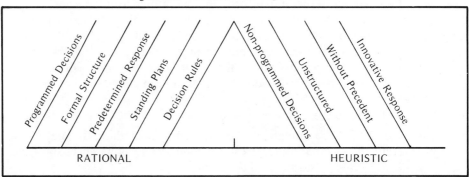

situations. You might already have a plan for the appropriate alternative to select should one of your employees become ill while on duty, or one for the use of a "prn" nurse to replace a staff member who is absent due to illness or vacation. Your only responsibility as decision maker is to respond to these routine problems by following the structured plan for such eventualities.

As we move from the highly structured, programmed end of the decision-making continuum to the less programmed, the problems become more unique and so the decision maker must be more innovative. At the extreme end of the continuum the decision maker has no precedent within the organization to rely on for guidance and the situation is completely new to him/her. In situations of this kind the decision maker may rely on intuition and an appeal to the supernatural.

Decision makers can and do employ a variety of methods for solving problems. These methods roughly correspond to the range of decisions on the continuum. The rational, logical, and objective approach to decision making tends to be at the programmed or *rational* end of the continuum while the methods that rely on intuition, subjective feelings, and innovation, are located closer to the unprogrammed or *heuristic* end.

In the real world of work the process of making relatively unprogrammed decisions is not a logically ordered progression toward the achievement of the ideal. It is, rather, a tortuous journey that involves interactions with people and concepts, and a shifting back and forth from the rational mode to the more intuitive and heuristic approach.[5]

Human decision makers, in contrast to machines, operate from two sets of premises: (1) *factual statements* about what can be proven to be true by empirical testing; and (2) *value statements* about what ought to be. In your interactions with people and ideas in the process of management, you rely on logic and common sense, and on your intuition, a feel for what is right and appropriate. Human decision makers such as yourself run into difficulty when they do not deal with the relevant information logically, or when they are not clear about their personal values in a decision-making situation. We will briefly discuss some common fallacies in thought patterns and then explore some relationships between values and decision making.

illogical or "crooked" thinking

One of the most frequently committed crimes of logic is seeing a cause-effect relationship that may not actually exist. This is done in either of two ways. You can *deny the antecedent* or you can *affirm the consequent*. In the first instance the false reasoning goes something like this:

If A is true, then B is true.
Therefore if A is false, then B is false.

This kind of faulty reasoning leads to poor decision making. For example, a head nurse might think: if we used Problem-Oriented Recordkeeping on our unit we would be able to document patient care more thoroughly. But we do not use POR on our unit, so we are not able to document patient care more thoroughly. The trouble with this line of reasoning is that although POR does facilitate documentation of patient care, the fact that it is not being used does not prevent the head nurse from trying to improve documentation on source-oriented records or some compromise between the two.

When a person *affirms the consequent*, the reasoning is as follows:

If A is true, then B is true.
Therefore if B is true, then A is true.

The most common incidents of this kind of reasoning are those in which people indulge in a kind of reverse reasoning in which they work backward to arrive at a conclusion that they *want to draw*. You should be particularly aware of this kind of illogical thinking when you are evaluating a decision that you have made. It may be true that you made the decision and that it had a favorable consequence or outcome. But the favorable outcome does not necessarily prove that your decision was a good one. Because of intervening circumstances the consequences could have been favorable for reasons other than the fact that you made a good decision. It is true that you made the decision, but the consequences may or may not have been the end result of your decision.

A third fallacy in thought patterns is *making overgeneralizations from specific instances*. This is a major hazard in appraisal of employee competence. It is such a common occurrence in so many different situations you probably have witnessed this kind of reasoning many times. Some examples might include:

- Some nurses who work in the operating room prefer not to have interpersonal relationships among themselves and patients; therefore all O.R. nurses prefer not to have interpersonal relationships.
- Mr. Santo has made several errors in charting vital signs on a graphic sheet; therefore Mr. Santo does not ever chart accurately.
- Nurse attendants usually do not have any formal education beyond high school; therefore all nurse attendants have not had formal education beyond high school.

Argument from analogy is another common mistake in logical thinking. It begins when one sees similarities between two situations. From this the person concludes that the situations share other similarities even though they may not. Analogies are fine up to a point, but they break down as a basis for argument when extended too far. For example, intuition plays an important role in making nursing decisions and managerial decisions, and so does knowledge of facts. Because of these similarities, one might try to infer that a person who is skillful in diagnosing nursing care problems will also be skillful in diagnosing management problems.

The fallacy in drawing this inference is that the basic knowledge needed to make sound nursing decisions is not exactly the same as that needed to make good managerial decisions. Nor are the values that influence each kind of decision precisely the same. Management of patient care in which there is direct involvement of the nurse is not the same as management of patient care indirectly through the efforts of others. To say that one who is highly competent in resolving patient care problems will also be highly competent in resolving management problems is an erroneous conclusion because it extends the analogy too far.

values and decision makers

The relationship of values to decision making has long been the concern of organization theorists. As we have said, the disciplines of philosophy and the social sciences have made significant contributions to the theory and practice of management and their efforts often have been focused on personal values and attitudes of individuals and the values of the organization.

The importance of values to the making of decisions seems rather obvious; explaining how values affect the decision maker, the process, and the acceptance or rejection of a decision is not quite so easy. In the final analysis a decision requires a commitment to an alternative. For the decisive leader or the decision maker who is working under pressures of time, there cannot be an endless search for information, ranking of preferences, and consideration of the consequences. Sooner or later a choice should be made. When there are two courses of action that seem equally reasonable and desirable, being more positive about your personal values helps reduce stress and conflict within yourself.

It is assumed that most of you have had experience in values clarification exercises in school or at continuing education programs. Those of you who are not familiar with the concept are encouraged to select some readings from the list of suggested readings at the end of this chapter. As a small sample of how you might clarify your values and give priorities to your objectives you might look at the following list of objectives. Choose the one that you value most, the one you would rank second, and so on to the lowest rank for fourth place.

"While on duty, I would like to have time to:
_____ eat lunch and take scheduled breaks."

_____ counsel employees who are not measuring up to standards.''

_____ teach employees who cannot competently perform some tasks.''

_____ plan for more delegation of duties.''

If you have difficulty ranking each of these activities from most desirable to least desirable, you can pair them and make a choice between only two, and then two others, and so forth. Using the list above, begin with the first item (taking breaks) and pair it with each of the others. Then take a second item and pair it with the remaining items (*underline your choice of each pair*).

> First pairing:
> *Taking breaks* vs. counseling
> *Taking breaks* vs. teaching
> *Taking breaks* vs. planning

> Second pairing:
> *Planning* vs. counseling
> *Planning* vs. teaching

Counting the number of times each activity has been underlined, you find that planning is your first priority and taking breaks second. You then assign either counseling or teaching third place and the remaining activity ranks fourth.

Values clarification requires time and effort when it is first begun. However, when you become surer and place more value on certain objectives, it is easier to state your preferences. It should go without saying that someone who places great value on particular activities and is committed to those values will benefit less from values clarification than will a person who is uncommitted and uncertain.

Perhaps it should be pointed out here that having very clear and highly valued objectives does not eliminate all uncertainty and risk in decision making. You can and must act decisively if you hope to be a leader, but you do so with the courage of your convictions and a willingness to accept responsibility for the consequences of the course of action you have chosen. Figure 4.2 is an exercise in values clarification that you might want to complete.

personal characteristics and decision modes

Effective decision makers, like effective leaders, exhibit some personal characteristics that are difficult to quantify but nonetheless are important to development of their own potential and that of their subordinates. Some

Directions: Rank each of the following according to your own personal preference. There are no right answers or correct order priorities. Using the number "1" as most desirable, and the number "10" as least desirable, indicate your order of ranking by placing a number in the space provided.

- Being popular with subordinates   _____

- Having respect of colleagues and peers   _____

- Being promoted to a higher level of management   _____

- Efficiently using time on duty   _____

- Being complimented by patients about the care received from my staff   _____

- Having favorable comments from physicians about the nursing care provided by my staff   _____

- Being complimented by managers of other departments about my cooperation   _____

- Having documented evidence of a high caliber of nursing care being provided to patients on my unit   _____

- Receiving an increase in salary without promotion to a higher level of management   _____

- Other (state in writing)   _____

figure 4.2   exercise in values clarification

observers have compiled rather extensive lists of personal traits common to people who make effective decisions. Most agree that these people are action-oriented and able to overcome inertia; they are sensitive to situations, innovative, and courageous.[6,7]

Additionally, effective decision makers are able to focus on the big picture. They view the organization as a whole and are aware of the part each subsystem and individual plays in accomplishing the mission of the organization. They can see the potential for achieving their own personal goals, the goals of their subordinates, and those of the organization. They are creative in finding ways to make these goals congruent.

In view of the many potentially conflicting elements in an organizational environment, it is not surprising that effective decision makers are those who can be flexible and adaptive. In organizations the *mode* of decision making typically is one in which the search for alternatives is limited.[8] The pressure of time and the limited supply of resources, both human and material, prevent the decision maker from searching until all possible alternatives identified and the best possible solution is found. As a kind of compromise, the decision maker uses what is called an *administrative or satisficing mode.*

When following this approach, the decision maker chooses the first alternative that he/she believes will meet the objectives set for resolution of the problem. If such an alternative is not found within a reasonable period of time, then the level of objectives is reduced and the first alternative that satisfies the new level of objectives is the one that is accepted. In short, the decision maker makes compromises and adaptations in the face of reality.

An example of the administrative, satisficing mode of decision making might be the actions of the head nurse who must provide adequate coverage for her patient care unit during a holiday weekend. Everyone would like to have the weekend off to spend with family and friends. The nurse-manager might want very much to give her staff members the time off and that could be one of her objectives, but she also is committed to providing quality care for her patients. It is apparent that both sets of objectives cannot be met because resources are limited. The head nurse cannot hire replacements for all of her staff members; the nursing office cannot provide her with relief nurses; and she cannot control admissions of patients to her unit and close it for the weekend.

In view of these and other realities of the situation, the head nurse simply does the best she can. And, having clarified in her own mind what is most important and what is of less value to her, she is better able to handle the conflict that invariably exists when all objectives cannot be met.

individual vs. group decision makers

In the resolution or alleviation of problems that significantly affect a group of people, there is the option of group decision making. Managers who are aware of the concept of group decisions in an organizational setting sometimes ask which approach is best: an autocratic mode in which the manager makes all the decisions, or a democratic style of leadership in which the members of the group engage in the process and make the final choice.

The question is based on two assumptions that are not necessarily true. First, that there are only two ways to provide leadership in decision-making situations, and secondly, that all such situations are pretty much the same. In response to these assumptions, decision theorists point out that there are several gradations between the extremes of autocratic and democratic leadership, and decision-making situations differ one from the other because of varying factors and conditions under which each decision is made.

As an example, we might look at the model for decision making developed by Vroom and Yetton. There are five decision methods that are available to the manager who is engaged in problem-solving activities. They have assigned each of these options a letter and a Roman numeral:

- Autocratic I (AI) — the leader makes the decision alone on the basis of information available to him/her.

- Autocratic II (AII) — the leader makes the decision; subordinates may or may not know what the problem is, but their role is to provide information that the leader uses to develop alternatives.

- Consultative I (CI) — the leader shares the problem with subordinates *individually*, requests their ideas and suggestions, and then makes a decision that may or may not be influenced by their input.

- Consultative II (CII) — the leader convenes the subordinates as a group, shares the problem, and obtains their ideas and suggestions. The leader then makes the decision that may or may not reflect their influence.

- Group II (GII) — The leader shares the problem with the group, coordinates their attempts at generating alternatives and forming a consensus, and accepts any solution that has the entire group's approval.[9]

The selection of one mode from the range of possibilities depends on the nature of the variables in a particular situation. These variables have to do with how well structured the problem is, how critical it is that group members accept the decision, whether their acceptance is essential to implementation, and their motivation to attain organizational goals, and the leader's skill in handling group conflict.

Models such as the Vroom-Yetton model for decision making and the Bailey-Claus model for decision making in nursing[10] are valuable tools for dealing with a complex task. They take a good bit of the risk and uncertainty out of decision making and allow for a more rational approach to the process. The reader is referred to the list of suggested readings at the end of this chapter for more information about these two models. In Chapter 6 we will discuss styles of leadership and the relationship of style to preference for individual and group decision making.

Decision making is an ongoing activity for managers. Some of you have more innate talent than others when it comes to using logic and intuition to arrive at a decision. But each of you can develop the potential that you do have by becoming more knowledgeable about trends in decision-making theory and courageously making the effort to put into practice the knowledge and skills that you already possess.

THE DECISION

The decisions that you make as a first-line manager will be evaluated by your superiors in terms of whether the decision objectives were met and the extent to which they contribute to the achievement of the mission and goals of the organization. From their perspective, the important criteria are the efficiency with which the decision was made and implemented and its effectiveness in preventing or resolving management problems.

Some evaluative questions that might be asked are:

*   Were the decision objectives (expected outcomes) clearly stated, measurable, easily communicated, and congruent with organizational objectives?
*   Were the expected outcomes realized fully, in part, or not at all?
*   Was the decision-making process efficiently utilized; that is, did the outcomes of the process justify the expenditure of time, personnel, and other resources?

Another criterion by which a decision might be evaluated is how well it is accepted by the people who must implement it. One can reasonably assume that people will work harder at accomplishing objectives that they consider valuable and worth working for. There will be times, however, when some members of the group will not be committed to the objectives and may not enthusiastically endorse them. This does not mean that the quality of a decision is necessarily poor. If a decision helps achieve important goals for your unit and for the organization, it can be considered a high-quality decision, even if it is not one that some group members fully accept.[11]

When you are faced with the dilemma of conflicting objectives and the means by which they can be achieved, you will need to apply your knowledge and skills in the management of conflict. This is discussed more fully in Chapter 9.

As stated earlier, the only decisions that can have totally predictable outcomes are those that can be totally programmed. Most of the decisions that you make will be only partly programmable; therefore, their outcomes will not be completely predictable. Because of intervening factors beyond your control, some of your decisions that seemed sound and rational at the time they were made may have less than desirable outcomes. William Morris notes that one should ask whether the decision maker could *reasonably* have chosen another alternative. If the answer is no, then the decision probably was a good one when it was made.[12]

REFERENCES

[1]A. H. Rubenstein and C. J. Haberstroh (eds.), *Some Theories of Organization*, (Homewood, Ill.: R. D. Irwin, Inc. and the Dorsey Press, 1966).

[2]J. Dewey, *How We Think*, (Boston: D. C. Heath & Co., 1910).

[3]D. Katz and R. L. Kahn, *The Social Psychology of Organizations*, (New York: John Wiley & Sons, 1966).

[4]J. G. March and H. Simon, *Organizations*, (New York: John Wiley & Sons, 1958).

[5]W. Gore, *Administrative Decision Making: A Heuristic Model*, (New York: John Wiley & Sons, 1964).

[6]P. R. Marvin, *Developing Decisions for Action*, (Homewood, Ill.: Dow Jones-Irwin, Inc., 1971).

[7]C. W. Emory and P. Niland, *Making Management Decisions*, (Boston: Houghton Mifflin Co., 1966).

[8]R. N. Cyert and J. G. March, *A Behavioral Theory of the Firm*, (Englewood Cliffs, N.J.: Prentice-Hall, 1963).

[9]V. H. Vroom and P. Yetton, *Leadership and Decision Making*, (Pittsburgh: University of Pittsburgh Press, 1973).

[10]J. T. Bailey and K. E. Claus, *Decision-Making in Nursing: Tools for Change*, (St. Louis: C. V. Mosby Co., 1975).

[11]N. R. F. Maier, *Problem-solving Discussions and Conferences: Leadership Methods and Skills*, (New York: McGraw-Hill, 1963).

[12]W. T. Morris, *Management for Action: Psychotechnical Decision Making*, (Reston, Va.: Reston Publishing Co., 1972).

SUGGESTED READINGS

J. T. Bailey and K. E. Claus, *Decision-Making in Nursing: Tools for Change*, (St. Louis: C. V. Mosby Co., 1975).

S. S. Coletta, "Values clarification in nursing," *American Journal of Nursing*, (Dec., 1978).

E. H. Erickson and Sister V. Borgmeyer, "Simulated decision-making experience via case analysis," *Journal of Nursing Administration*, (May, 1979).

W. C. Gill, "Lowering decision levels," *Supervisor Nurse*, (Oct., 1974).

E. LaMonica and F. Finch, "Managerial decision making," *Journal of Nursing Administration*, (May-June, 1977).

K. A. Mahon and M. D. Fowler, "Moral development and decision making," *Nursing Clinics of North America*, (March, 1979).

A. Marriner, "The decision-making process," *Supervisor Nurse*, (Feb., 1977).

A. Marriner, "Behavioral aspects of decision making," *Supervisor Nurse*, (March, 1977).

J. F. Schweiger, "The indecisive leader," *Supervisor Nurse*, (Nov., 1978).

B. S. Simon et al., *Values Clarification: A Handbook of Practical Strategies for Teachers and Students,* (New York: Hart Pub. Co. 1972).

A. G. Taylor, "Decision making in nursing: An analytic approach," *Journal of Nursing Administration*, (Nov., 1978).

D. B. Uustal, "Values clarification: application to practice," *American Journal of Nursing*, (Dec., 1978).

V. H. Vroom, "Decision making and the leadership process," *Journal of Contemporary Business*, (Autumn, 1974).

chapter 5
index

chapter
motivation

INTRODUCTION

Managers in every kind of organizational setting and at every level of administration share the opinion that one of the most troublesome and puzzling aspects of their job is motivation of personnel. Throughout the history of management, organizational theorists and practicing managers have searched for resolution of the problem. The result has been an abundance of theories, some conflicting, some impractical, and some that are still in the developmental stage.

There is not now, and probably never will be, a single theory of motivation that will provide managers with all of the guidelines needed to improve performance, relieve apathy, and increase efficiency and effectiveness. The needs, wants, and expectations of people at work are but one set of variables to be considered in a study of the complex and dynamic psychosocial-technical system that is the organization. One must also take into account the interpersonal interactions of individuals and groups, the organizational structure and climate and the goals and aspirations of the organizational systems.

Having said all this to prepare you for the study of motivation and to give you some appreciation of its complexity, we will now look at the problem of motivation with a more positive attitude. The work of theorists and practitioners can be helpful to you by providing some insight into the nature of the problem and some practical suggestions for improving performance through techniques of motivation.

In this chapter we will discuss the concepts of job satisfaction and productivity; their interrelationships in an organizational system; and some approaches to improving the level of both in a health care setting. Another concept that will be covered is that of job enrichment and the use of motivators that are focused on the work itself. Finally, we will attempt to apply some principles of current motivation theory to the practice of management and give you some insight into the influence of managers in creating a working environment that is conducive to job satisfaction, job enrichment, and productivity.

KEY CONCEPTS IN MOTIVATION THEORY

Since the time of the industrial revolution managers and theorists have been concerned with the concepts of *job satisfaction* and *productivity*. It seems reasonable to assume that greater employee satisfaction automatically results in improvements in the total operation of the organization, that is, in the quantity and quality of work produced by the workers. However, a causal relationship between the two has *not* yet been established.

job satisfaction and motivation

Job satisfaction is an elusive term. There is no precise definition that is universally accepted by theorists, practicing managers, and people at work. One of the most frequently quoted definitions is the one suggested by Price: "The degree to which members of a social system have a positive affective orientation to membership in the system."[1] In short, if people feel good about belonging to a work group in an organization, they are believed to be satisfied with their jobs.

Price's definition reflects the humanists' view of people as goal-directed and social beings whose attitudes shape their motives. Hence, motivation comes from within the person. Motive forces based on feelings and values lead to behavior that is directed toward the goal of satisfying a need.[2] The task of motivation theorists is to identify the motivating forces that lead to satisfaction of the needs of people at work, which in turn, it is assumed, will lead to higher levels of productivity.

In the historical development of motivation theory, the traditional view of man as an economic being gave rise to the belief that money was the most important, if not the sole, motivator.

economic incentives

During the early history of organization theory it was believed that motivation was simply a matter of providing an external incentive. The approach was basically that of the "carrot and the stick." Motivation was thought to come from outside a person. Stimulation took the form of reward for work well done and punishment for failure to measure up to the expectations of superiors in the organization. The literature of that time reflected the belief that people had an *inherent* need for money and that wages (the carrot) provided the means for satisfying that need.[3]

Modern theorists certainly recognize the importance of wages as a major factor in job satisfaction, but they do not see money as a primary motive force. An external reward such as money does provide incentive and reinforcement, but rewards provide the *means* by which some needs can be satisfied, for example, food, warmth, and the housing needed for adequate rest. In this age of relative affluence, however, many people in the highly developed industrial countries have needs and goals beyond those that can be satisfied by the expenditure of money.

As a salaried employee you can appreciate the importance of wages as a major component of job satisfaction. As a manager you also should be concerned with the fairness and equity of wages paid to subordinates. Humanistic theorists have no quarrel with the notion that economic reward is important to job satisfaction. They do, however, question the assumption that money is an effective *motivator*. In the real world, experience has shown them to be correct.

For example, the paying of time-and-a-half for overtime has not motivated people to work more efficiently, as could be expected if money were an effective motivator. In fact, experience has shown that overtime pay can have the opposite effect. If a person desires more money in his/her paycheck, he/she can accomplish this by working more slowly and collecting overtime pay. In effect, money has the potential for motivating people *not* to work efficiently.

Another factor to consider in regard to monetary rewards and motivation is an employee's perception of the fairness with which money is exchanged for work done. If people feel that they are being paid a wage that is not commensurate with the amount of work they do, they will be motivated to reduce their effort, take the maximum time allotted for sick leave, etc., or quit their jobs. This could have significance for you in terms of absenteeism, poor work habits, and attitudes of resentment among the lower paid personnel on your staff.

While there may not be much that you can do about increasing the salary of your subordinates, you can create opportunities for them to receive rewards other than a monetary one. There is no doubt that many of these people work very hard and expend much physical energy in the performance of their assigned tasks. Recognizing and expressing appreciation for the contributions they make toward accomplishing the goal of quality patient care can help bridge the gap between what they believe their work to be worth and the pay they receive for the work they do.

This leads us to a review of the other variables that are thought to be important to job satisfaction and productivity.

other components of job satisfaction

In the 1950's the work of Maslow, Herzberg, and other need theorists gave impetus to research efforts to identify specific factors that contribute to the satisfaction of people at work. The broader view includes the dimensions of *opportunity for promotion, level of achievement, role and status, recognition, authority,* and *autonomy*.

In their study of job satisfaction with workers in medical settings Slavitt et al. identified six components of job satisfaction that seemed most relevant to the type of occupations found in health care organizations. These components are:

* *pay*, including dollar remuneration and fringe benefits;
* *autonomy*, or the amount of job-related independence, initiative and freedom either permitted or required in daily work activities;
* *task requirements*
* *organization requirements*; that is, constraints or limits imposed on job activities by organization structure;
* opportunities for formal and informal *social contact* during working hours;
* *job prestige/status*, which is defined as the overall importance or significance felt about the job at both the personal and organizational level.[4]

These and similar components of job satisfaction are based on humanistic theories of motivation. In order to understand how these views evolved, we will digress for a moment and review the major contributions to motivation theory and researchers' attempts to show relationships between human needs, motivation, and productivity. We will begin by discussing the importance of productivity and its dimensions in a health care setting.

productivity

The output of workers is a legitimate concern of the administrators of an organization. An organizational system does not survive for very long if it does not meet environmental demands for the products and services it is expected to provide. In a highly technical system productivity is focused on the efficient cost-effective performance of men and machines. The goal is a profitable return on the organization's investment of resources. The productivity of the organization is evaluated in terms of economic gain and other tangible measurements of the ratio of input and output.

Because of the kinds and scope of services demanded of an organization in the health care delivery system, managers in organizations of this type need a broader definition of productivity. This broader concept would, according to Bennett, encompass *attitude* as well as "purely economic and tangible measurement of output per manhour and machine hour."[5]

The notion of total output as the sum of measurable outcome of task performance plus attitudes of workers toward the care and service they provide implies an appreciation of the values held by workers and their psychosocial needs and goals. A series of studies conducted in 1927 were among the first experiments that gave empirical evidence of the fallacy of the assumption that labor is a commodity to be bought and sold. These studies, called the "Hawthorne experiments" called into question the effectiveness of manipulating external rewards of wages and hours to keep employees marginally satisfied and to motivate them to achieve the goals of the organization.

the Hawthorne experiments

The experiments were conducted over a period of five years at the Hawthorne Works of the Western Electric Co. in Cicero, Illinois. They involved thousands of hours and scores of researchers, yet the concept was relatively simple. It started with a group of six females whose job was the assembly of a telephone relay. For a period of almost a year these women worked in a room where their working conditions could be carefully controlled, their output measured, and their work closely observed.

Changes were made in the women's hours, wages, rest periods, organization of work, and the degree of supervision by and consultation with their superiors. Physical changes in their working environment also were made over a period of time. There were no correlations found between these changes and productivity. Variations in temperature, humidity of the room, etc. had no measurable effect. However, with the introduction of each variable related to *social conditions* production kept increasing.

The social variables were exemplified by frequent interviews with the women during which their opinions, hopes, and fears were eagerly sought by the researchers. They were questioned in a nonthreatening way, sometimes in their supervisor's office, about their working conditions. They were allowed to set their own production quotas. Their physical health and well-being were of great concern to the investigators. In essence, the women who once had been typical workers performing a routine job with little or no attention from management, had become very important persons.

Researchers later realized that they had created what became known as the "Hawthorne effect," that is, the special attention given to the workers during the study had contaminated the experiment and clouded determination of the effectiveness of each variable. But one thing did become clear. Human relations among workers and their managers played an important part in formation of an *esprit de corps* and this was directly related to an increase in output. No longer could management contend that optimum productivity was solely a function of fair wages and adequate working conditions.[6]

implications for managers. The findings of the Hawthorne experiments and similar studies have the following implications for you as a first-line manager:

- *Challenge* team members to do their best; work at convincing them that theirs is a winning team.

- Listen to gripes and complaints, but *avoid consoling* subordinates and thereby giving them the impression that they are to be pitied for the amount of work expected of them by higher levels of management and administration.

- Be *loyal* to the organization for which you work, and expect the same loyalty from your subordinates.

- Create opportunities for subordinates to *accept responsibility* for setting goals and devising ways to achieve them.

- Work for the well-being of the *whole group*, not for the happiness of particular individuals or subgroups.

- Maintain an interest in both *people* and *task performance*.

- Recognize the strength of *informal work groups* based on sentiments and feelings of group members. Status and social interaction in groups of this kind can have a significant effect on the productivity of individual group members. Try to direct the influence of informal groups into constructive rather than destructive channels.

HUMAN NEEDS AND MOTIVATION

The Hawthorne studies marked a transition from traditional management thought to the humanist era of organizational theory. Humanists view people as unique individuals who are goal-directed; that is, human behavior is directed toward *goals* that *satisfy needs*.

Theorists recognize two general kinds of human need: *inherent* or inherited needs and *learned* needs. The first broad classification includes the primary or *physiologic* drives or needs that are essential to the survival of the individual and procreation of the species. The second category includes the secondary or social needs that are learned as part of the socialization process.

Probably you are familiar with Maslow's hierarchy of needs and its application in the nursing process. According to his classification, the basic *physiologic needs* include a need to be free from fear of deprivation, danger, and threat at work as well as away from it. The next level of needs, in ascending order, are the *social needs* to belong to a group, and to be accepted by and liked by others; *egotistic needs* of self-respect, and respect and recognition from others; finally, the *need for self-actualization*, that is, "the desire to become everything one is capable of becoming."[7]

NEEDS FOR ACHIEVEMENT AND AFFILIATION

David McClelland, in collaboration with J. W. Atkinson, constructed a theory derived from Maslow's hierarchy and focused on the need for achievement and the need for affiliation in an organizational setting. They contend that there are three major relevant motives at work in an employment situation: (1) the need to strive to succeed, and to excel when measured against a standard (achievement); (2) the need for warm and friendly relations (*affiliation*); and (3) the need to influence the behavior of others, that is, to be in *control*.[8]

McClelland makes the interesting suggestion that motivation for achievement is learned by the individual through cues picked up in his environment from earliest childhood through young adulthood. He believes that the motivational level of young people can be raised by conditioning them to seek the "ideal self" which represents what they want to be and think they should be. Aspirations to succeed can be raised by conditioning a person to have high expectations for himself/herself.

In your dealings with your subordinates you will have frequent opportunities to "condition" them to think of themselves as achievers and to help them capitalize on their need to achieve. An important prerequisite to guiding a person to the achievement of personal and organizational goals is knowledge of the person as a unique individual.

Each of your subordinates has his/her own special abilities, talents, likes, and dislikes, and potential for growth. Diversity is both a delight and a challenge to the nurse and the nurse-manager. You would not think of preparing a nursing care plan without any idea of the nursing care needs of your patient. Neither can you devise a plan for motivation of an employee without knowing something of his/her personal attributes, preferences, hopes, and aspirations.

The kinds of information that could be helpful in determining effective ways to satisfy an employee's needs for achievement and affiliation might include:

- Career goals
- Educational background, including courses (credit and noncredit) that are *not* related to nursing
- Work experience and avocational interests, hobbies, etc. *not* directly related to nursing
- Special aspects of his/her work that he/she finds most rewarding

- Tasks that are most difficult to perform and those he/she can do with ease
- Co-workers who contribute to the enjoyment of his/her work
- Age and sex of patients he/she prefers working with
- Specific patient care problems that he/she finds challenging and those likely to cause emotional stress. For example, if a relative has died from severe burn injuries, it may be difficult for him/her to care for a burn patient.

Much of McClelland's work was with people in management positions. Through his studies he identified some characteristics that he believes to be typical of managers who are highly motivated by a need for achievement. At this point it might be interesting for you to try a little self-analysis and measure your own perceived traits with those of McClelland's managers. The characteristics that he identified have to do with decision making and a desire for growth and achievement of personal goals.[9] They are as follows:

- Tendency to initiate the decision-making process
- Desire to take upon yourself responsibility for making decisions and a willingness to accept responsibility for their results
- Willingness to take moderate risks in order to achieve excellence
- Desire for feedback on results of your decisions and actions. Feedback need not always be complimentary: you are able to listen to and act on suggestions for improvement.
- Desire to expend energy and work hard to accomplish your goals

job enrichment

The idea of job enrichment has been around since the early days of management science when practicing managers and writers in the Human Relations Era saw the need for making work more meaningful and satisfying. In the early 1960's Herzberg and his associates added to the basic concept some conclusions drawn from an analysis of both the individual and the organizational environment.[10] Herzberg suggested that satisfaction and dissatisfaction are not two ends of the same continuum; hence, reducing dissatisfaction will not increase satisfaction. He viewed them as two separate sets of factors in regard to the motivation of workers. (See Figure 5.1).

Herzberg believed that improving salary, working conditions, and other "hygiene" factors would reduce dissatisfaction among workers, but that such improvements in the environment would not reduce apathy and

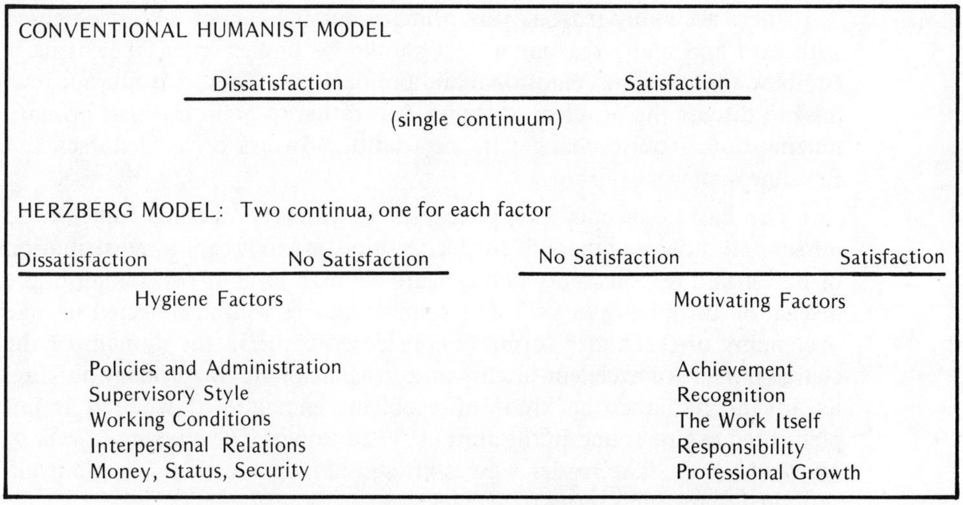

```
CONVENTIONAL HUMANIST MODEL

        Dissatisfaction                            Satisfaction
                        (single continuum)


HERZBERG MODEL:  Two continua, one for each factor

Dissatisfaction          No Satisfaction      No Satisfaction          Satisfaction

        Hygiene Factors                          Motivating Factors


    Policies and Administration              Achievement
    Supervisory Style                        Recognition
    Working Conditions                       The Work Itself
    Interpersonal Relations                  Responsibility
    Money, Status, Security                  Professional Growth
```

figure 5.1   Herzberg's two-factor theory of motivation

conflict. In order to do that, motivators related to finding satisfaction in *the work itself* would have to be employed.

Job enrichment is a management strategy for change. It is, therefore, a highly complex system of techniques that involve significant changes throughout an organization particularly in regard to the division of work and the appraisal of performance.

The process of job enrichment focuses on the work itself. Its major goals are (1) making the work more meaningful; (2) structuring tasks so that workers believe they are personally accountable for the outcomes of their efforts; and (3) providing an appraisal system that gives the workers knowledge of the outcomes of their work on a regular basis.

In recent years nursing literature has been filled with writings about ways and means by which the task of nursing can be made more meaningful, nurses can become more responsible for the outcomes of nursing, achieve more autonomy, and deal with the issue of accountability. One of the most frequently suggested means to accomplish the goals of job enrichment for nurses is through a change from a function-team nursing system of work division to primary nursing.

However, the "ideal" of primary nursing is far from the reality of work division in most health care agencies. There is ample evidence to support the belief that a continuous one-to-one nurse-patient relationship provides greater job satisfaction and opportunities for job enrichment among professional nurses.[11] The question is not whether it would enrich the job of nurses but whether hospital administrators and other top-level managers in the health care system see it as the best means for achieving organizational goals.

There are many reasons why primary nursing cannot be implemented with ease and many reasons why it should be implemented. The issue is complex and often has emotional and political overtones. It is not our purpose to discuss the problem at length, but rather to point out that primary nursing does require changes in the traditional roles of head nurses and first-line managers.

The basic concepts and principles of primary nursing forces head nurses and other members of the leadership staff to accept a redistribution of power and responsibility and a relatively high level of risk taking in the delegation of nursing tasks.[12] The primary nurses will be expected to take over many of the duties formerly considered to be in the domain of the charge nurse. An excellent discussion of the rationale for primary nursing, its advantages, and the kinds of problems encountered when it is implemented can be found in the June, 1977 edition of *The Nursing Clinics of North America*. The reader who is interested in pursuing this topic is encouraged to read this series of articles.

For those of you who are working as head nurse or charge nurse in a conventional setting in which functional and team nursing are the models in use, the following suggestions for attaining the goals of job enrichment are offered:

- Utilize the principles of management by objectives (MBO) to help your subordinates set goals, receive feedback on performance, and participate in preparing unit goals for achievement of organizational goals.

- Assess the level of competence of each staff member, including professional and technical nurses, and base their assignments on competence, compatibility of patient needs, and opportunity for growth in the job.

- Assign each patient to a particular staff member from the time of admission to the day of discharge so that, insofar as possible, there will be a continuous nurse-patient relationship.

- Be willing to live with some risk taking in the delegation of responsibility for patient care.

- Provide opportunities for group participation in scheduling work and determining how the work will be done and by whom.

- Whenever possible combine components of the nursing task to form new and larger modules of work. Problem-oriented record keeping facilitates this by permitting the formation of work modules around a group of nursing care problems.

- Implement a formal employee appraisal program (see Chapter 10).

SOME APPLICATIONS OF MOTIVATION THEORY

Richard Steers and Lyman Porter offer some practical suggestions for using current motivation theory to improve employee performance and contribute to job satisfaction and productivity.[13] Among their suggestions are: (1) managers must initiate changes that bring about more positive work attitudes and a better motivational climate, and (2) managers should have a clear view of themselves, their own motives, strengths, and weaknesses. We will take the first of these suggestions and discuss some of the ways you can develop more positive attitudes in your subordinates and provide a work environment conducive to higher levels of performance.

managers must make it happen

So many times the failure of employees to perform as expected is blamed on "poor attitude." Nurse-managers seem to feel that if their subordinates would only have the right attitude toward their work, there would be no need to worry about trying to motivate them. This assumption is partly right and partly wrong.

Attitudes, motives, and behavior are interrelated. Attitudes arise from values and are strengthened or reinforced through positive feedback via communication and social pressure. Undesirable attitudes are weakened or extinguished by negative feedback, that is, ignoring the unacceptable behavior that is a manifestation of the attitude. Figure 5.2 shows the cyclic nature of the relationships among attitudes, motives, behavior, and feedback. It is, of course, an oversimplification of a very complex concept, but it may help you develop some planned and purposeful techniques to improve performance.

To begin with, you may need to develop a more positive attitude toward the problem. Many managers seem to be convinced that nothing can be done to change what they perceive to be poor attitudes. We hear such statements as, "They just don't care," or, "They don't take their work seriously," and "They are lazy and irresponsible." All of these assumptions are based on observed behavior. People who "don't care" *do something* that gives the impression of not caring. Perhaps they ignore call lights, give a haphazard bed bath, drag their feet when giving medication for pain, or in some way behave in a manner that is undesirable.

Each of these examples of unsatisfactory attitude manifested by overt behavior can be dealt with in a positive and meaningful way. It may be that environmental conditions are contributing to poor attitudes and the apparent lack of motivation to meet acceptable standards of performance.

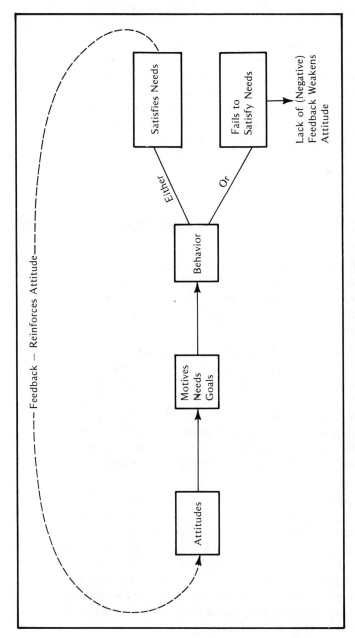

figure 5.2 relationships of attitudes, motives, behavior

environment and motivation

Mager and Pipe, in their analysis of performance problems, identify some environmental elements that may be responsible for the poor attitudes and behaviors that managers find so exasperating. They recommend that anyone wanting to improve the performance of a subordinate might achieve his goal by changing the *conditions* or *consequences* responsible for nonperformance. Four such conditions common to situations in which there is evidence of lack of motivation to perform efficiently and effectively are: (1) It is punishing to perform as desired; (2) Nonperformance is rewarding; (3) It makes no difference whether or not performance is desired; and (4) There are obstacles to performing as desired.[14] We will take each of these conditions and give examples of the kinds of activities that might be responsible for poor performance.

punishing to perform

How many times have you seen a new employee work very hard for the first few weeks or months of employment, completing assignments ahead of time and eagerly volunteering to help others? After a while there is a gradual slowing down and eventually she seems to adjust her pace to the level of others on the staff or maybe "goof off" even more than the others. What happened to her enthusiasm and eagerness?

There could be any number of things going on that contribute to her loss of motivation to work hard. Has the head nurse given her extra work because she was so efficient and able to handle it? Are other members of her team taking advantage of her willingness to work hard, exploiting her eagerness to help so that they do not need to work as hard as they could? Is she being ridiculed by other staff members who use her but do not respect her diligence? Are cynical remarks being made about a new broom sweeping clean? Are there subtle, or maybe not so subtle, remarks suggesting that she will settle down once she knows the ropes?

The nurse-manager who is aware of this kind of "conditioning" of an employee whose performance is declining should do some detective work to find out what is going on. No amount of prodding, teaching, or threatening from the head nurse is going to make any difference to an employee who is being punished for working hard.

nonperformance is rewarding

Rewards for nonperformance might come from the manager as well as from the nonperforming subordinate's peers. As an example of the nurse-manager being the dispenser of rewards for failure to meet expectations, consider the attention given an employee who is chronically late for work.

The employee blames her frequent tardiness on family problems. The children get sick, the car breaks down, her husband is visiting his sick mother, and on and on. Each time she is late the head nurse spends at least 5 or 10 minutes listening to the employee's explanations as to why she is tardy. She hears her out, commiserates with her, and does her best not to lose her temper. The head nurse doesn't want to appear heartless, the woman does have problems, and so she takes even more time during the day to counsel the employee and try to help her work through her problems.

At some point the head nurse should take a good hard look at what is happening here. Certainly she wants to express an interest in the personal problems of her employees, but does she really want to accept the role of social worker and personal psychologist in addition to her other roles? How much of her time is she spending *reinforcing* the employee's undesirable behavior? What about her obligations to other employees and her patients?

Employees can reward one another for nonperformance in countless ways. This usually happens when a wholesome team spirit is lacking and some kind of perverse pride is taken in seeing how little work they can get by with. Usually there is a ring leader in the group, encouraging the others to slow down and take it easy. There are two strategies the nurse-manager might use to deal with this kind of situation.

First, identify the ring leader and try to change her behavior. Give positive feedback for things that she does well and provide opportunities for her to exercise her leadership abilities in a more productive way. Or, reprimand her for the work she is not doing and threaten her with demotion or firing if she doesn't improve. If she is a very strong leader and is able to influence the other group members, attempts to reprimand her may backfire.

Using positive reinforcement is the ideal alternative. Social psychologists recommend ignoring undesirable behavior (giving *negative* feedback is giving *no* feedback) and rewarding desirable behavior. The problem with this approach is that the nurse-manager must decide how much undesirable behavior he can tolerate before the welfare of her patients is jeopardized.

The second strategy in dealing with the overall situation is to reward the good behavior of everyone in the group, including the one who is suspected of being the ring leader. Compliment them for work well done and broadcast the good news to persons outside the group so that those who perform well will experience increased status and esteem because of their competence and diligence.

it makes no difference

In the third type of situation that might be responsible for nonperformance, the employee *gets no feedback* on her performance, nor does she get any for nonperformance. It just doesn't seem to matter to anyone whether she does a good job or a poor one.

The evaluating function of management is presented in more detail in Chapter 10. We have already discussed the importance of knowledge of results as a major contributor to job enrichment, and the evaluator role of the manager. All of this information is relevant to motivation of employees.

obstacles to performing as desired

An obstacle can be something present in the path to accomplishment of a goal, or a gap in the road that must be bridged. In the case of a frustrating obstacle, it might be that there is too much work to be done by the number of people available or that there are too many distractions in the environment. Examples include too many visitors in a patient's room, too many nonnursing personnel attending to the patient throughout the day, too many people in the nurses' station reading and writing on the charts.

In some hospitals and clinics a lack of sufficient supplies can be an obstacle to performance. Sometimes this can be remedied rather easily. In one extended care facility the charge nurse noticed that the patients' temperatures were not being taken and recorded according to policy. When she checked with the nurse attendants she found that the patients' personal thermometers, issued to them at the time of admission, were not on their bedside tables. The elderly patients, having been assured that the thermometers were their very own, hid them safely away in their purses, cigar boxes, and other remembered and forgotten places. It was not lack of motivation on the part of the nurse attendants, as the charge nurse originally thought, but rather a lack of readily available thermometers. The problem was resolved by rounding up all of the thermometers and replacing those that were lost, labelling each with a patient's name, and storing them in the medicine room next to the nurses' station.

Inadequacy of staff, inaccessibility of equipment, and poor organization of the unit can have a negative impact on the motivation of workers. If their leader is apathetic, doesn't efficiently organize the work and see to it that employees have the tools they need to get the work done, productivity and job satisfaction will be low. Employees look around and see in their environment signs of disinterest on the part of management. This tells them, in effect, that their jobs can't be too important.

In each of the four situations identified by Mager and Pipe as being common conditions responsible for nonperformance, the remedy usually is less difficult than the diagnosis. Nurse-managers hoping to improve employee performance need to develop their analytic skills to find out what is going on in any given situation. Then they use their knowledge of behavior modification to reinforce desirable behavior and eliminate that which is less desirable.

"know thyself"

Returning to the previously mentioned suggestions of Porter and Steers, we see that self-analysis is essential to the growth of the manager and ultimately to improvement in the work situation. Certain old sayings were attributed to the figures known as the *seven sages*. Among those sayings was the advice to know yourself. Before we can begin to understand what is going on in the minds and hearts of others we must confront our own strengths and weaknesses, motives and desires. We learn about ourselves through self-analysis and soul searching and through information we get from others who see us from an entirely different perspective.

During a management class conducted for head nurses and supervisors a young nurse-manager took on an assignment in self-discovery. She was working as night supervisor in a small rural hospital in which she first began as a nurse attendant during high school. She completed a course in practical nursing and worked at the same hospital as an LPN. Later she went back to school to become an RN and completed her degree in nursing.

As part of her project she listed the things that she felt had motivated her to continue her education and to work for promotion from staff nurse to charge nurse and eventually to supervisor. Having a fairly good idea of her own strengths and weaknesses as *she* saw them after this exercise, she then proceeded to seek input from those who had worked with her through the years and were now under her supervision.

Many of these people had once been in a position to teach and guide her and to work with her as a peer and colleague. She asked them to list, anonymously of course, the things she did as a supervisor that they liked and behaviors that annoyed them. It took a great deal of courage for her to do that because she was feeling insecure and frustrated in her job. She had serious doubts as to whether she really was capable of doing the job well, considering the circumstances in which she was working.

When she gave her report to the class she was very honest in her appraisal of herself and admitted surprise that the people who now worked under her supervision were strongly in favor of her *acting like a supervisor* when at work, making decisions that were for the good of everyone, upholding her standards, and treating everyone equally. They felt this way even though many of them socialized with her when off duty. The most satisfying outcome of the project was, in her words, "finding out I'm OK, I'm a pretty good supervisor and I can be even better if I will just go ahead and do the things I know I should do, and try to do them as fairly and honestly as I can."

Self-analysis should be a creative endeavor. It provides the means by which you can set goals, develop your potential, and become more self-actualizing. It also is an exercise in honesty. It helps you to accept yourself as you are, and that is the first step toward becoming what you hope to be. Accepting yourself with full knowledge of your strengths and weaknesses is a prerequisite to accepting others and helping them grow in their jobs.

REFERENCES

[1] J. Price, *Handbook of Organizational Measurement*, (Lexington, Mass.: D. C. Heath & Co., 1973).

[2] T. Haiman, W. G. Scott and P. E. Connor, *Managing the Modern Organization*, (Boston: Houghton Mifflin Co., 1978).

[3] F. Taylor, *Principles of Scientific Management*, (New York: Harper and Bros. Pub., 1911).

[4] D. B. Slavitt, et al., "Nurses' satisfaction with their work situation," *Nursing Research*, (March-April, 1978).

[5] A. C. Bennett, "Employee motivation: The key to improved productivity," *Hospital Topics*, (Feb. 1972).

[6] E. Mayo, *The Human Problems of an Industrial Civilization*, (New York: The Macmillan Co., 1933).

[7] A. Maslow, *Motivation and Personality*, (New York: Harper and Row, 1954).

[8] D. McClelland, *The Achieving Society*, (Princeton, N.J.: Van Nostrand, 1961).

[9] D. McClelland and D. H. Winter, *Maintaining Economic Achievement*, (New York: Free Press, 1962).

[10] F. Herzberg, *Work and the Nature of Man*, (New York: World Publishing Co., 1966).

[11] G. Marram, et al., *Primary Nursing*, (St. Louis: C. V. Mosby Co., 1974).

[12]E. H. Elpern, "Structural and organizational supports for primary nursing," *Nursing Clinics of North America*, (June, 1977).

[13]R. Steers and L. Porter, *Motivations and Work Behavior*, (New York: McGraw-Hill, 1975).

[14]R. Mager and P. Pipe, *Analyzing Performance Problems*, (Los Angeles: Fearon Pub. Inc., 1970).

SUGGESTED READINGS

S. Axne et al., "Staff motivation through a self-help design," *Supervisor Nurse*. (Oct., 1976).

R. L. Bunning, "Changing employees' attitudes," *Supervisor Nurse*, (May, 1976).

A. Chopra, "Motivation in task-oriented groups," *Journal of Nursing Administration*, (Jan.-Feb., 1973).

S. Cooper, "Committees that work," *Journal of Housing Administration*, (Jan.-Feb., 1973).

R. Fleishman, "Human resources motivation," *Supervisor Nurse*, (Nov., 1978).

W. L. and J. M. Ganong, "Motivation and innovation: Concerns for nursing administration," *Journal of Nursing Administration*, (Sept.-Oct., 1973).

W. L. and J. M. Ganong, "Motive force: A key to evaluating nurse managers," *Journal of Nursing Administration*, (July-Aug., 1974).

D. L. Howell and W. R. Boxx, "Motivating workers on routine jobs," *Supervisor Nurse*, (May, 1973).

A. Levenstein, "Alienation in the hospital," *Supervisor Nurse*, (May, 1975).

J. Lysaught, "No carrots, no sticks: Motivation in nursing," *Journal of Nursing Administration*, (Sept.-Oct., 1972).

A. Marriner, "Motivation of personnel," *Supervisor Nurse*, (Oct., 1976).

_____. *Primary Nursing: Nursing Clinics of North America*, (Philadelphia: W. B. Saunders Co., June, 1977).

chapter 6
index

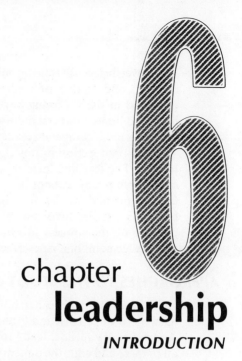

chapter
leadership

INTRODUCTION

Nursing and management literature is replete with writings that point out the need for strong and effective leadership among practitioners and suggest ways in which that need can best be filled. For centuries theorists have tried to isolate the components of leadership and integrate them into a general theory that will tell us what effective leadership is, how an individual can become an effective leader, and criteria that can be used for selection of people for leadership positions.

Theorists and practicing managers and administrators no longer ponder the question of whether leaders are born with the necessary personal characteristics and motivation, or if it is a matter of teaching them the techniques and tools they need to be successful leaders. They realize that the leader is a product of both his/her inheritance and environment and that leadership is best understood when placed in the context of a given situation. A person is an effective leader when there is a favorable combination of all the elements contained within the situation.

In this chapter we will discuss the "nature" and "nurture" approaches to the study of leadership and then proceed to the more recent situational theories that have evolved from trait theory and behavior theory. An individual's personality certainly influences his/her behavior, but that behavior, in turn, depends in part on the circumstances at any given moment, day, or week. The application of theories to actual practice in the work setting is not, and probably never will be, a matter of applying a mathematical formula to the resolution of a management problem. Human nature and human behavior have a way of defying precise measurement and the establishment of universal standards. Secondly, no two management problems are exactly the same.

Nevertheless, practicing managers can utilize current and traditional concepts and models of leadership to improve their skills. The material presented in the following pages is offered in the belief that even a very basic and limited understanding of these concepts and models can help you become a more competent leader.

The final section of this chapter is focused on the role of the leader as teacher. The teaching-learning process is interwoven throughout the fabric of leadership. One cannot be a leader without being a teacher, even if only by example and emulation. Planned and purposeful teaching is described here as a process involving both the teacher and the learner. The components of the process are briefly explained and examples of activities within each component described.

APPROACHES TO THE STUDY OF LEADERSHIP

The efforts of leadership theorists have been focused on finding answers to three basic questions: *Who* is a leader? *What* does a leader do? And *how* does a leader lead? In recent years a fourth question incorporates all of these and adds the dimension of *where* leadership is taking place.

Trait theory, one of the oldest and most traditional approaches, seeks to answer the first question. In the 1950's behavioral scientists began to develop a *behavior theory* that set aside personal characteristics and concentrated on the functional aspects of leadership. Through observation of leaders and analysis of accounts of leadership in action, they addressed the question of what a leader does.

Out of answers to the question, "How does a leader lead?" evolved a description of the manner in which a leader tries to influence the behavior of others. A *leadership style* combines the leader's personality traits, values and attitudes, and is manifested by overt behavior that is characteristic of a particular style.

Style theory, in turn has led to the *situational approach*, which considers relationships between traits of the leader, requirements and objectives of the particular situation in which leadership is taking place, the values, attitudes, and needs of those being led, and the organizational variables that might affect the situation.

Although the basic concepts of trait theory and behavioral theory of leadership probably are not new to you, we will begin with a brief overview of these theories and then go on to the newer theories that have evolved from them and attempt to show how these theories are applied to the practice of management.

trait theory

Trait theory is the oldest of the theories of leadership. It evolved from philosophical debates over the personal attributes of "great men" in society, and centered on the task of finding relationships between personality and successful leadership.[1] Through decades of social science research, theorists have observed and read accounts of successful leaders and compiled lists of their personal traits. Because of the complexity of the problem, a pattern or "profile" of the kind of person who could be expected to lead effectively in all kinds of situations has yet to emerge.

One aspect of leadership that has received considerable attention is the question of ethics. It might be assumed that a "good" leader is one who serves well the needs of the groups and of society as a whole. But when we look at such political leaders as Adolph Hitler and such religious leaders as Jim Jones of Guyana, we are brought to the realization that a sick society or group can choose to follow a sick leader.[2] Probably you have seen firsthand some examples of employees following a leader, appointed or otherwise, who encourages them to behave in a manner that is destructive to themselves and harmful to the people around them.

The failure of trait theorists to develop a model by which specific personal attributes can be perfectly correlated with success in leadership does not necessarily detract from the significance of their contribution to a fuller understanding of the concept of leadership. The absence of a model prevents one from making accurate predictions about the success with which a certain type of person will be able to lead, but the characteristics identified by trait theorists as desirable in a leader can be useful to you as a guide for self-analysis and the setting of goals for improvement.

The following list developed by Ghiselli is representative of the kinds of characteristics thought to be correlated with success in management.[3] These are:

- *Intelligence.* An above average intelligence is desirable, but if there is too great a distance between the intellectual capacity of the leader and the general level of intelligence of the followers, the leader becomes less effective, possibly because of problems of communication and difficulty in understanding one another's viewpoint.

- *Supervisory skill.* This includes interpersonal skills and ability to establish rapport with subordinates.

- *Initiative.* This encompasses both the ability to act without stimulation from anyone else, and to perceive existing problems or foresee those to come.

- *Self-assurance.* Such a characteristic is similar to confidence and related to the ability to cope with stress. Leaders who can concentrate their attention on issues despite environmental distractions are usually more effective, as are those who can think about more than one thing at a time.

- *Individuality*. The possession of a pattern of traits different from others in the situation. In effect, the leader stands out in a crowd.

Personality is the essence of a person, the sum total of his/her inheritance, cultural and religious background, life experiences, prejudices and biases, hopes and aspirations. From the viewpoint of the humanists a person is always in the process of becoming something more than he/she already is. It is difficult to change a person's total personality; difficult, but not impossible.

Signs of personal growth in your job as manager are signs of personality change; not in a pathologic sense, of course, but in the sense that the attitudes, values, and opinions that are the foundations of personal attributes have changed. Developing your strengths, and strengthening your weaknesses as a leader is a continuous process that begins with self-evaluation. Evaluation requires the comparison of your individual traits with those that trait theorists have found helpful in the effective leadership of others. The results of their work can be useful to you in determining how you can either change your attitudes and behavior, if that is what you want to do, or accept yourself as you are at this time of your life and look for situations for which you are better suited.

behavior theory and styles of leadership

Behaviorists are concerned with the overt actions of management leaders when engaged in the functions of planning, organizing, directing, and controlling. Figure 6.1 shows a continuum of leadership behavior ranging from an autocratic, boss-centered style to the democratic, subordinate-centered style. It is the classic model developed by Tannenbaum and Schmidt to portray the range of styles used by leaders in decision-making situations.

Other models show slightly different classifications. For purposes of our discussion we use a classification that divides styles of management into five categories: *autocratic, bureaucratic, participative (which is subdivided into democratic and consultative) and free-rein.* We will briefly discuss each style and list some of the relative advantages and disadvantages of each. Bear in mind that the descriptions are admittedly oversimplified and are presented only to give you some idea of the options one has and probability of success in using a particular style in a given situation.

autocratic: Behaviors in this category range from those of the stereotypical top sargeant, "do-as-I-say-or-else" style, to the paternalistic "father knows best." Either way, the subordinates have precious little freedom and no opportunity to participate in problem solving and decision making.

The autocratic or authoritarian style may be appropriate in an emergency or crisis situation. It is the quickest and most efficient way to get

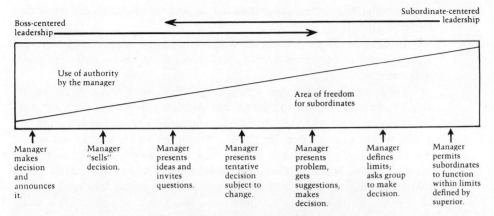

figure 6.1 Tannenbaum's "continuum of leadership behavior"

things moving and doesn't leave much doubt about who is to do what, and when and how it is to be done.

A motherly or fatherly style is helpful when a subordinate has a low tolerance for ambiguity, is immature, and insecure. The problem with this approach is that it dooms the subordinate to perpetual immaturity and insecurity because it does not allow for personal growth and development of potential.

Another disadvantage is that it places great responsibility on the leader and demands that he/she be competent and knowledgeable in every case and at all times. If such expertise is lacking in the leader (and it inevitably is in at least a few areas of performance), the one-way communication that is typical of this style will make it very difficult for the leader to become aware of his/her personal shortcomings. The results can be disastrous in terms of loss of resources, including human lives, in a health care organization as well as on a battlefield.

bureaucratic: When a leader uses this style the subordinates are told what to do. Not because the "boss says so," but because the "book says so." Procedures and policy manuals, rules and regulations, the sticks and bricks of organizational structure, are the main support of the bureaucrat.

This style does have the advantage of guaranteeing consistency in the performance of procedures, in treatment of personnel in regard to days off, working hours, salary, and so on, and in setting standards for appraisal of employee performance. Its disadvantages are that there is no recourse when common sense dictates that there should be an exception to the rule. If the rules are ambiguous, as they tend to be in large and complex organizations, then productivity decreases, morale is low, and subordinates are frustrated and resentful.

In Chapter 9, we discuss the disadvantages of bureaucratic attitudes and the conflict that arises when professionals are given no leeway to make judgments.

participative: The leader who is comfortable with this style of leadership allows subordinates to take part in problem solving and decision making. The *democratic* participative leader encourages group participation and abides by the group's decision. The *consultative* leader acts as you would expect a consultant to behave; that is, the group is aware of the problem and offers suggestions for its resolution, but the leader makes the final decision. (Note: You may recall that in Vroom and Yetton's model for decision making mentioned in Chapter 4, there were two levels of consultative style. These two levels roughly correspond to the democratic and consultative styles of participative leadership in this classification.)

A major advantage of a participative style of leadership is the commitment people feel toward implementation of a decision they have helped to make. A problem that is shared becomes "our" problem. Other advantages are the opportunities for releasing creativity and developing the potential of subordinates. There are strong motive forces at work when a participative style of management is used.

The major disadvantage, however, is the amount of time it takes and the possibility that the process may not result in the desirable goals of efficiency and effectiveness. Sometimes pressures from within the group produce a watered-down version of the original goals and objectives of the leader and group. This style demands a strong and alert leader who can regain control when necessary.

free-rein: When a leader uses this style it does not mean that he/she exercises absolutely no control over the group. That is *laissez faire*, or "anything goes." The leader who uses a free-rein style does set the goal to be achieved and declares the rules of the game, for example, the constraints on time and other resources. He/she then becomes accessible to the group for guidance and clarification when they feel a need for help.

This style allows for full utilization of the talents and energies of the group members who have been delegated full responsibility for problem solving. There is, however, a high level of risk. The leader must have a thorough knowledge of the level of competence and personal integrity of the group members.

Theorists who have developed classifications of leadership style do not suggest that there is a one best style. While it is important that a leader choose a style with which he/she is comfortable, that is not to say that the preferred style is always the most appropriate. Flexibility implies a willingness to move back and forth along the continuum of styles, plus a reasonable level of skill in utilizing a variety of styles. Later, when we discuss situational leadership theory, we will see that it may be necessary to substitute another leader so that there is a better matching of variables in a particular leadership situation.

leadership style and orientation of the leader

Analysis of the two extremes of the leadership continuum led to further study of their relationship to one another and attempts to develop a mathematical model for leadership behavior. In the 1950's, studies at Ohio State University led to the concept of these two styles as two separate variables, the *product* of which is leadership behavior.[4,5] Figure 6.2 shows the two variables on a style analysis graph.

Autocratic leaders are believed to be concerned with structure, that is, the nature of the *task* and how it is to be done by group members. Democratic leaders, on the other hand, emphasize *consideration* for the group members. The two dimensions of concern for task or productivity and concern for people became the basis for further study. Because of the complexity of human interaction in the production of goods and services, the two variables subsequently were broken down into smaller elements and presented on a grid. One of the best known of these is the managerial grid developed by Blake and Mouton.[6]

A model that seems to have more relevance to the practice of management is that devised by Paul Hersey and Kenneth H. Blanchard and called a

figure 6.2   two variables on a style analysis graph

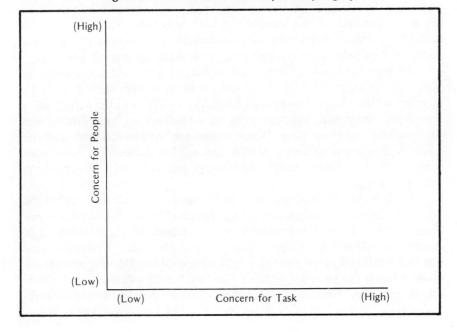

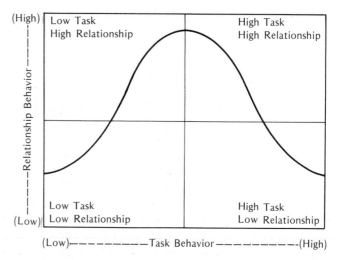

figure 6.3   Hersey and Blanchard's four styles of leadership model

Tri-Dimension Leadership Effectiveness model. The three dimensions under consideration are: (1) the task vs. relationship behavior of the leader; (2) the environment in which the leader is functioning; and (3) the maturity of the group members.

The task and relationship behavior of the leaders combine to form four basic styles of leadership (see Figure 6.3). *Task behavior* is defined as the extent to which the leader is likely to organize and define the relationships between him/herself and the members of the group (followers). It is closer to the autocratic end of the leadership style continuum. The task-oriented leader is concerned with establishing organizational structure, giving directions, setting deadlines, and supervising the activities of subordinates.

Relationship behavior is defined as the extent to which the leader is likely to maintain personal relationships between him/herself and the members of the group. This group of behaviors is closer to the participative end of the continuum. The leader provides feedback to the followers and encourages input from them. There is two-way communication, and the leader is an effective listener as well as sender of messages. The leader provides positive reinforcement for motivation and seeks ways to enrich the jobs of subordinates.

A self-evaluation tool prepared by Hersey and Blanchard is called the Leader Effectiveness Adaptability Description (LEAD). As the name implies, it helps the leader determine his/her adaptability or flexibility in choosing a style of leadership appropriate to the situation. The instrument was first published in the February 1974 edition of the *Training and Development Journal* in an article entitled "So You Want to Know Your Leadership Style?" Another source is an article entitled "A Look at Your Supervisory Style," published in the June, 1976 issue of *Supervisor Nurse*. If you are interested in having an opportunity to get some insight into your own leadership style and how it either changes or remains the same in a variety of situations, the LEAD instrument is recommended for independent study or in a workshop or classroom setting.

style theory and situational theory combined

The Hersey and Blanchard model of leadership theory[7] represents the current trend toward combining the concepts and techniques of style theory with those of situational theory in hopes of developing a comprehensive theory that can be applied to a variety of managerial situations. One of the most interesting and potentially useful models is Fred Fiedler's "Contingency Model of Leadership Effectiveness."[8]

Fiedler's model can provide some helpful insights into the leadership role of nurse-managers. Much of what you do as a leader is done intuitively. If you have been fairly successful in leading your subordinates in the accomplishment of goals it is probably because you have a good grasp of the whole task, yet you may not be totally aware of each of the various elements that make up the whole. By learning about the results of analysis of the total phenomenon of leadership, you will be better able to isolate some knowledge and skills that you can implement with competence and some in which you need improvement.

Fiedler's model represents a *quantitative* approach to the measurement of variables in any given leadership situation. He has devised three scales which represent each of the three major components of the leadership role. These major components and their corresponding scales are:

- *Component:* The leader's interpersonal relationships with members of the group and the relationships among group members.

  Scale: *Leader-Member Relations Scale*

- *Component:* Degree of structure in the task to be performed by the group.

  Scale: *Task Structure Rating Scale*

- *Component:* Formal authority of the leader

  Scale: *Position Power Rating Scale*

The total score for the three scales is the Situational Control Scale. In assigning values to each scale, Fiedler attaches greatest importance to leader-member relations.

Whereas other theorists have given equal weight to concern for people and concern for tasks, Fiedler contends that the better the relationships among group members and between leader and group, the stronger the impact of leadership.[9] Leadership requires a willingness on the part of people to be led in the accomplishment of goals. If they do not see the goals as valuable or if they are not willing to be influenced by another person, that person will not be able to lead them effectively.

Before going on to further discussion of Fiedler's contingency model and situational leadership theory, we will digress for a moment and clarify some concepts basic to situational theory. These are: *power, influence,* and *control.*

the relationships of power, influence, and control

Power has to do with the continuous give and take that goes on in any leadership situation that is alive and well. Votaw[10] points out that it is difficult to think objectively about power because subjective and emotion-laden ideas about "good," "evil," "freedom," and "justice" have themselves been closely intermingled with the notion of power. He then goes on to give three assumptions characteristic of modern concepts of power:

1.   That power has both a positive and a negative side; though subject to abuse and corruption, it can be useful in resolving problems of a society.

2.   That power is essentially an interpersonal relationship that is reciprocal in nature. A person or group is permitted to have power because of certain attitudes and expectations held by the person or group granting the power.

3.   That power, like wealth, is constantly being produced and consumed. There is no *static* quantity of power.

Influence is a subtle force operating outside the person or group who are the followers. The leader *indirectly* affects the behavior of others through influence. Yurah and Walsh suggest that strategies for influence may be based on advice, suggestions, persuasion, or propagandizing. Or the leader can use power with "sensitivity, knowledge, and humaneness to affect the behavior of others."[11]

Control is another concept that has emotional overtones and potential for abuse. In a democratic society, control might imply a loss of freedom and an inability of followers to make decisions that affect them. Modern concepts of control suggest a benevolent and humanistic approach to the exercise of control. The purposes for which a leader uses control are expected to be centered on the achievement of goals that are important to and beneficial for the followers as well as for the leader and the organization.

The successful leader has situational control only when attention has been paid to interpersonal relationships and to structuring of the task to the extent that those who must perform the task will be able to do so competently. As manager, one of your main functions is controlling. You will be able to carry out the many activities inherent in this function if you can use your strategies for influence and sources of power to best advantage.

sources of power. *Authority* is defined as legitimate power to influence others. The persons who are being influenced recognize the power of the leader as appropriate because of that person's position in the organizational structure. But authority is not the only source of power available to a leader. French and Raven[12] have identified a total of five sources of power that should be of interest to you in the understanding and application of leadership theory. The sources of power are:

- *Legitimate power:* potential for influence that is derived from being in a position of authority. For example, having been appointed head nurse, charge nurse, or team leader, you are recognized by other members of the staff as having some power to direct and control the activities of employees working under you.

- *Referrent power:* also called *affection* power. It is the potential for influence that comes from being liked or respected by members of the group. Research indicates that having the respect and affection of the group makes the leader more influential than he/she would be without the ability to make others like him/her.

   Some authorities separate respect from affection, pointing out that it is possible for a leader to be respected even though group members do not necessarily like him/her. This is an important point to remember because managers sometimes make the mistake of trying to be well liked and "popular" with the group. In their attempt to be liked by everyone they could lose the respect of some members and therefore reduce their power to influence them.

   Some theorists go even further and suggest that some managers are able to exert influence because they provide a moral example that others want to follow.

- *Expert power:* the potential for influence that derives from the leader's having the skills and expertise needed or valued by the group. When a leader is competent in the performance of tasks that are difficult or require special knowledge and skills, he/she is better able to give support and guidance to those working toward a common goal.

If members of a group see someone other than the leader as having more expertise in the performance of a task, the appointed leader will lose some expert power; it has been shifted to the person having the requisite knowledge or skills. This may happen in a situation in which a specialist such as a respiratory therapist participates in planning and implementing a care plan for a patient suffering from respiratory distress. You should not feel threatened by the diminishing of your expert power in this area. Many of the people in the allied health occupations are knowledgeable and skilled in a specific task. Such specific skills should not be generalized and applied to all other nursing and management situations.

One of the greatest mistakes a nurse-manager can make is to try to be all things to all people. This reflects an autocratic mentality and leadership style. You only set yourself up for frustration and failure if you expect to be the only person who can and should have power to influence your subordinates. It is more sensible to recognize the expertise of others and to use it to best advantage to accomplish the goals that you value.

- *Reward power:* also called monetary power because its source is the ability to dispense or withhold money, recognition, and other objects valued by group members. As first-line manager you may have only limited influence in this area if you have no voice in decisions about pay increases and promotion of employees who have demonstrated improvement. If you avoid the responsibility for systematically evaluating the performance of your subordinates, and want no part of recommending them for advancement, special awards, and other symbols of recognition for work well done, then you relinquish some of your reward power.

- *Coercive power:* the potential for influence which is derived from the ability to impose or withhold punishment. It is the other side of the reward power coin. The most obvious coercive power is physical force such as that used by crime overlords when they make an offer "you can't refuse." For the nurse manager the coercion might come, directly or indirectly by recommendation, from the ability to fire, demote, or suspend without pay an employee whose behavior is unacceptable.

    Coercive power should be used only as a last resort because it can have many social and psychological effects on the member being punished as well as on other members of the group. It is a crude way to handle a delicate situation and can easily backfire, destroying the effectiveness of other sources of power. If a group is subjected to coercive power, the result may be the forming of a strong bond among group members. They may begin to actively or passively oppose the leader and eventually undermine her position to the point that she is, in effect, no longer their leader.

APPLICATION OF THEORY TO PRACTICE

Situation theory and models of leadership provide some useful tools and techniques for effective leadership strategies. We have barely scratched the surface in the preceding discussions and explanations of these theories and models. You will need to continue to develop and deepen your understanding of leadership theory and gain experience in its practical application in the world of work. The strategies of a theory are learned by applying them. It is through this effort that you become more familiar with a theory and eventually grasp it in its totality. Once you have done this, you will be able to modify it and apply it to meeting your own needs.[13]

Fiedler's situation theory is based on the assumption that the variables of leader-member relations, task structure, and position power can be altered so that they more nearly fit the leadership style of the leader. It is believed that changing personal leadership traits in the leader is far more difficult and time consuming than changing the other variables in a given situation. If the other variables cannot be changed to the extent that they should be, then it may be necessary to substitute another leader with a more compatible style until the task is accomplished.

Altering elements within each variable of a given situation requires that the leader be skillful in using effectively the tools and techniques of planned and purposeful change. The process of change and the collaborative relationships between the person who makes the change and the person or persons who are the clients are discussed in Chapter 8.

changing leader-member relations

The factors within the variable of leader-member relations have to do with how well the leader gets along with the members of the group, how effectively group members can function as a team, and the psychosocial atmosphere in which all of these people are working. A friendly and helpful atmosphere may be difficult to measure, but there is no question that it has a powerful influence on the satisfactory accomplishment of tasks.

Change is essential to improvement of any situation. Yet whenever there is change there is going to be some friction and conflict. If conflict already exists in leader-member relations it will be amplified and aggravated by attempts to introduce new ideas and tasks. When there is too much conflict the goals of the proposed change will not be reached. On the other hand, the complete absence of conflict is symptomatic of complacency and a lack of awareness of the need for doing things differently. The status quo is preserved because "that's the way we have always done it." Healthy leader-member relations indicate the successful management of conflict, not its avoidance or suppression. The topic of conflict management is discussed in Chapter 9.

A leader has several alternatives to changing the leader-member relations variable. If he/she is a low-task, high-relationship type of leader, it could be that he/she should *not* alter the leader-member relations variable but should change the task-structure instead. A low-relationship, high-task leader is not going to score well on relationships with subordinates. Such a person will need to appraise his/her personal attitudes toward people in general and group members in particular, perhaps question his/her Theory-X assumptions about human nature and work toward the goal of moving closer to the Theory-Y end of McGregor's continuum.

Group members also should be evaluated in terms of how well they get along with one another. Their ability or inability to do the job certainly influences their willingness to cooperate. Remember that each of the variables in the situation affects the other. It may be that changing the degree to which the task is structured by adding more detailed guidelines and instructions will improve their competence and self-confidence and thereby improve their ability to work as a team. Changing task structure will be discussed shortly.

Changing people's attitudes toward their leader and one another is, of course, far more difficult and complicated than changing task structure. It is always easier to deal with things than to deal with people. If a particular task objective must be accomplished in a given period of time, it may be easier to change the nature of the group by changing the relative positions of individuals in the group so that the deadline can be met.

To illustrate this point we will consider a situation in which the objective is to improve documentation of nursing care on nurses' notes and progress records. Nurses A and B are not adept at writing notes and they see no point in "writing down everything we do." Their feeling is that it is more important to meet the nursing needs of the patient than to meet the needs of administrators who are concerned with the auditing of charts and accreditation. No amount of persuasion and discussion can convince them that clear and concise documentation contributes to the quality of care patients receive.

In contrast, nurses C and D are skillful in charting their patients' progress, and they enjoy the challenge of documentation and nursing audits as a technique for evaluating the quality of care patients receive. In this particular situation it might be more effective or productive to rearrange the assignment mode so that the nurses who do not want to document patient care must report to the nurses who do. This means, of course, that nurses A and B will work under the direction of nurses C and D who could function as module leaders or as team leaders. They would then be responsible for coordinating and documenting the care given by the two who have not shown a willingness to accept that responsibility. There is a possibility, that after a while, nurses A and B will change their attitudes because they see the value of documentation and its relationship to the nursing process.

A rather drastic measure that could be necessary to change leader-member relations is to either transfer, demote or fire one or more members who are identified as foot-draggers or trouble-makers or both. The leader will need to verify any suspicions that he/she has about particular individuals in the group and validate those suspicions before making such a recommendation. Again, we can see how the variables are interrelated and interdependent. Hiring, firing, and other similar measures are related to the leader's position power.

CHANGING TASK STRUCTURE

The structure of a task is measured according to the degree to which each of the following factors is present or absent:

1. A clearly stated goal; that is, a detailed description of the finished product or service, or someone who can provide such a description.
2. A step-by-step procedure to follow in performance of the task and a standard that is recognized as the best way to perform the task;
3. A one, best solution to the problem or an ideal outcome for the task;
4. An easy way by which one can check to see that the task was done right, and a chance for the leader and the group to find out how well they have done in time to improve in the future.

Nursing procedures are highly structured tasks. Those that are less structured usually have to do with initiating and implementing concepts and changes in the way broader goals and objectives are accomplished. For example, an unstructured task could be the introduction of a system by which staff members decide how coverage will be provided and accept responsibility for assigning days off, covering for one another during vacation and illness, and so forth. Another unstructured task might be the objective of utilizing a problem-oriented system of record keeping in a patient care unit. Tasks such as these can be structured, of course, but the structure of the task is more individualistic because it has different requirements in different situations. Nursing procedures can be structured and written in a procedure manual for use in a variety of settings. Implementing a primary nursing approach in a hospital's surgical unit is not the same as implementing it in an intensive care unit where the approach to nursing care probably is more like primary nursing than functional nursing.

Fiedler suggests three ways by which tasks can be structured so that overall situational control is improved: (1) by training; (2) by developing procedures, policies, and other criteria and standards, and by giving feedback on *meeting the criteria* rather than on *"trying" or being cooperative*; and (3) by gaining experience in performance of the task.[14]

It is apparent that a leader who is task-oriented would be much happier structuring the task than would one who is more concerned with interpersonal relationships. Task-oriented leaders handle very difficult and very easy tasks more easily than do high-relationship leaders. If immediate results are needed, it is the task-oriented leader who can be the most effective leader. If you recall the behavior of the leader who prefers a more auto-cratic style of leadership, you will see why a task-oriented leader is more likely to get immediate results when the situation calls for quick and efficient action.

changing the leader's position power

The variable of position power on Fiedler's model is related to the leader's sources of legitimate and expert power. If the leader is not in the position of head nurse, supervisor, or other recognized place on the organizational chart, his/her legitimate power is either very weak or nonexistent. If he/she cannot recommend hiring and promoting, firing or demoting, or has no means by which to confer other rewards and punishments, then his/her reward power is low.

This is of importance to the beginning head nurse who may not be aware that the bureaucratic structure of the organization in which he/she is working may be responsible for a loss of legitimate and reward power. In most health care organizations the bureaucratic structure is slow to change. The anger and frustration of professional nurses in highly structured organizations is reflected in current literature, in formal debate and informal discussions.

An alternative that many head nurses have chosen when confronted with the problem of weakened legitimate power is to turn to sources of affection power and expert power. An example of strengthening one's power base by strengthening expert power is a head nurse who is relatively new in her position. Because of inexperience and self-acknowledged personal insecurity, she does not have a high level of reward power. She does not feel confident of her ability to evaluate the performance of her subordinates and has not taken part in the organization's employee appraisal program long enough to be able to evaluate their performance objectively and make recommendations.

The head nurse is asked by the director of nursing to implement a change requiring the use of a flow sheet for charting routine care. The task is one with which the head nurse is quite familiar. She has had experience in using a flow sheet and can use one competently. She also is able to teach the task to her subordinates without difficulty. Her expert power in this particular situation helps make up for her weakness in legitimate and reward power.

application of situational theory

The following example is presented to demonstrate some of the concepts and techniques that have been previously discussed. It is not intended to show how all of the variables in the situation can be altered, nor is it a comprehensive example of situational and trait theory. It is meant as a stimulus to the reader to delve deeper into the subject and to attempt to apply what we have learned from leadership theorists.

leader-member relations and position power

Mrs. Locke, head nurse, has the affection and respect of her staff members. On the Hersey-Blanchard model her style of leadership would fall into the high-relationship and low-task category.[15] On the Fiedler Member Relations Scale she probably would have a high score.

Because of her lack of training and experience in regard to the task to be performed, she would have less control due to loss of expert power. This would be compensated for to some extent by the fact that she does evaluate the performance of her subordinates; has an official title of authority, and can recommend promotion, demotion, hiring, and firing (reward and coercive power).

task structure

The task is to initiate and implement modular nursing on Mrs. Locke's patient care unit. This would involve a change in the way in which duties and responsibilities of the various staff members are assigned. The director of nursing has asked Mrs. Locke to try modular nursing on her unit as a pilot project. Eventually she hopes to use it throughout the hospital.

Mrs. Locke, being more person-oriented than task-oriented, was less concerned with details of the task than with how her staff would accept the change. She consulted with them and asked their input into the decisions to try modular nursing on their unit. In spite of some misgivings about how it would work and what effect it would have on them, the group members agreed to try it. They reasoned that if it didn't work no harm would be done and nobody could say they didn't give it a chance.

Their *maturity level* for this task would not be high because they had no training or experience in performing this particular task. Additionally, they were not committed to making the project a success and thus were not setting a very high standard for achievement. Risk taking was at a low level because they felt that failure would not necessarily reflect imcompetence on their part, and they were more dependent on a reward system consisting primarily of compliments for being cooperative and easy to get along with.

Not being aware of all of these negative influences and low level of situational control, Mrs. Locke was surprised and disappointed when the attempt at instituting modular nursing on her unit was a disastrous failure. She had hoped that her affection power was strong enough to ensure cooperation and competence from her staff members.

The director of nursing very quickly became aware of the inability of the head nurse and her staff to perform the task. She had at her disposal a consultant who recommended that the task be more structured and the head nurse be replaced as leader for this task until she and her group gained task maturity. The person chosen as leader for the performance of the task was a member of the Department of Staff Development who had knowledge of and experience in using modular nursing for assignment of duties and responsibilities. She structured the task by preparing detailed instructions on how the assignments were to be made, advantages and disadvantages of modular nursing, and its basic concepts and rationale for using it. During the first two weeks she actually made the assignments and met frequently with the group members and head nurse to determine how well the new approach was working. Together they evaluated their performance and devised plans for improvement of their competence level.

As the group matured and Mrs. Locke gained expertise and experience, the temporary leader gradually withdrew her support and decreased her participation. Mrs. Locke's style of leadership, bolstered by the substitute leader's shift to a high task-behavior style until the task became easier, was ideal for long term maintenance of task performance by her staff.

These concepts and tools for determining and changing variables in a situation can be used for many tasks that are the responsibility of a nurse-manager and her employees. Leadership is complex; it is a dynamic process that can lead to growth and development of both the leader and the followers if handled in a systematic and knowledgeable manner.

LEADERSHIP AND THE TEACHER ROLE

If you were to ask a group of nurse-managers where they would place the teacher role in a list of priorities and preferred duties and responsibilities, chances are that most of them would put it near the bottom of the list. And yet, if you were to observe these same nurse-managers at work, probably you would see many of them teaching and working with their employees to help them learn more and develop their potential. Teaching, like nursing, is a very broad, generic term that is difficult to define and delineate. It does not necessarily mean formal classroom instruction conducted at specified times. Teaching and learning can take place anywhere, at any time and in an unlimited number of ways.

There are some compelling reasons why a nurse-manager should develop expertise in the area of teaching. First, to recall previous discussions of the definitions of management, the goal of management is the development of people, the releasing of internal motive forces to the end that employees grow in their jobs and become more self-actualized persons. Second, by training staff members and improving their level of task performance, the nurse-manager increases the job maturity of group members.

This maturity factor is an important variable in leadership situations. In the role of teacher the nurse-manager has opportunities to strengthen his/her expert power and referent power. And, finally, training is one of the leader's options for changing task structure to a more favorable level for situational control.

It should be noted that we are talking about training in the performance of specific tasks related to nursing. Not all teaching is the same, and in some instances it may be more appropriate for teaching responsibilities to be assumed by the Department of Staff Development. For example, the more general kinds of information and skills needed by every employee probably could be taught more efficiently by a centralized in-service education department. This might include cardiopulmonary resuscitation, fire drills, preparation for disasters, general orientation to the agency's personnel policies, and less specialized procedures.

There are, however, some tasks that require specialized knowledge and skills on the part of employees working in a particular patient care unit. These are best taught as decentralized in-service education conducted in the work setting. It is a more individualized and personalized kind of training that meets the more immediate needs of employees and improves their performance of specific tasks.

teaching adults

Most of us think of teaching and learning as two separate entities taking place in a traditional classroom setting that is highly structured. The teacher is the source of information, the fountain of knowledge, and the dispenser of grades. The students sit before the teacher, a captive audience waiting to "be taught." But this is not really what teaching and learning are all about. They represent a process involving partnership and mutual respect and cooperation. The teacher is a guide and a facilitator of learning, but in a sense everyone in the group is teaching and learning. This can only happen in a relaxed, nonthreatening environment in which everyone is free to make suggestions, ask questions, and discover answers without fear of reprimand or ridicule.

This approach to teaching and learning is particularly important to adult learners who may have some very negative feelings about classrooms and teachers. Because they did not have many successful learning experiences in their childhood and young adulthood, they feel inadequate and fearful about "book learning." It is important that adults be given a sense of dignity and self-worth while they are learning and that they have opportunities to contribute their talents, skills, and creativity during the teaching-learning process.

Malcolm Knowles, an authority on adult education, presents some interesting assumptions about changes that take place as a person matures, and offers some helpful suggestions about their implications for teachers of adults. According to Knowles, as a person matures, (1) he perceives himself more as a self-directing human being and less as a dependent personality; (2) he accumulates a growing reservoir of experience that becomes a useful resource for learning; (3) his readiness to learn becomes more oriented to the developmental tasks of his social roles; and (4) his time perspective changes from one of postponed application of knowledge to immediacy of application.[16]

If adults perceive themselves as being more self-directed, it behooves the teacher of adults to work toward helping adult learners determine their own learning needs and to avoid telling them what they need to learn. Adults learn more easily if they are actively involved in selecting learning objectives and, using their reservoir of experience, are able to participate in decisions about how these objectives might best be achieved.

Because adults are more concerned with immediacy of application, they learn more readily when they are convinced that the material they are studying has practical application in their everyday duties and responsibilities. The nurse-manager functioning in the teacher role can take advantage of this concern for relevance and applicability and recognize it as a motivating force for reaching learning objectives.

Readiness to learn is essential to the success of a teaching-learning activity. Adults learn in a series of plateaus rather than in a continuous upward progress. It is almost as if they need time to slow down a little and assimilate new knowledge and practice new skills before moving on to another level. This should be understood by both teacher and learner so that neither will become discouraged by an apparent lack of progress and motivation. During these periods of leveling off, employees and manager can attend to other duties and responsibilities without feeling guilty and they can become more relaxed about teaching and learning.

Not all adults have had learning experiences in which they were consulted about their learning needs, asked to share responsibility for their learning, and encouraged to engage in self-directed learning activities. For those who were taught in the traditional way, it is often a shock to find out that they are expected to do something more than passively receive instruction. Their initial reaction to a partnership kind of teaching may be one of resistance and frustration. It takes time for them to realize that the ''you teach and I learn'' style of instruction is not the kind of teacher-learner relationship that is thought to be most productive for adults. Once the initial shock and dismay are overcome, the adult learner usually experiences a sense of release of motivating forces and a vastly improved self-concept.

What we have been talking about here is a decentralized, personalized kind of in-service education or on-the-job training that involves interaction between the teacher and the learner in a released, nonthreatening environment. The key words are interaction and environment; they are the basic ingredients of the learning experience.

the teaching-learning process

The process of teaching and learning has four major components: diagnosis of learning needs, planning, instruction, and evaluation. In each phase of the process both teacher and learner are actively involved, and the role of each tends to merge with the other and reverse positions. In other words, the teacher becomes the learner and the learner is the teacher. The outcome of the teaching-learning process is personal growth and a fuller realization of the potential of the people involved.

If you have ever taught anyone in a systematic and purposeful way, you know that once you become engaged in the process you become painfully aware of your own learning needs. A clear, concise, and detailed explanation of the subject matter demands a thorough analysis of the content and a synthesis of the knowledge you have gained during the analysis. Analysis is a breaking down of the subject to find relationships among its elements. Synthesis is a restructuring of these elements in your own way so that you can present it according to your understanding of the relationships and inferences drawn during analysis.

In the process of teaching and learning there are three domains in which the activities can take place: cognitive, psychomotor, and affective. If you are not familiar with these, they are easily remembered as head, hands, and heart. Figure 6.4 presents a brief summary of these domains of learning.

diagnosis of learning needs

During this phase the teacher and learner work together to detect differences between the learner's current level of performance and the desired level. The major activities in this phase are: (1) establishing criteria that state in objective and measurable terms what the competent person knows and is able to do willingly and with care when performing specific tasts; (2) assessing the learner's current status in respect to these criteria or goals; and, (3) identifying learning objectives that will help the learner meet the criteria or goals.

Learning objectives should be measurable and realistic in terms of what the learner can reasonably be expected to accomplish. Behaviorists contend that learning can only be considered to have occurred when there is a change in behavior; it is performance and *not* the person that is being appraised. This is a key concept that cannot be ignored throughout the entire process. It allows for more objective evaluation, and centers on the learner's ability to demonstrate a certain level of knowledge, skill, and attitude. If there is no change in behavior, there is no evidence that learning has taken place, no matter how carefully instruction has been planned and implemented or how diligently the learner may have studied and practiced.

Type of Behavioral Objective	Most Appropriate Techniques
COGNITIVE DOMAIN *Knowledge and comprehension* of factual information, principles, and generalizations, recall of experiences, etc.	Lecture, television, debate, dialogue, interview, slide film, book-based discussion, case method, reading, critical incident process, demonstration, audience.
PSYCHOMOTOR DOMAIN *Manual skills.* New ways of performing.	Skill practice exercise, drill, coaching, demonstration and return demonstration, role playing, question and answer.
AFFECTIVE DOMAIN *Attitudes.* Adoption of new feeling through experiencing greater success than with old: *Values.* Adoption and priority arrangement of beliefs; *Interests.* Satisfying exposure to new activities.	Experience-sharing discussion, role playing, case method, television, lecture (sermon), debate, dialogue, slide film, dramatization, guided discussion. Values clarification techniques.

*Adapted from Malcom S. Knowles, The Modern Practice of Adult Education, 1st ed., Exhibit 76, p. 294.

figure 6.4   matching techniques to desired behavioral outcomes

As an example, we can take the task of caring for a patient undergoing peritoneal dialysis. Objectives should be written using active verbs describing what a person is able to do when performing the task competently. The objectives are learner-centered; that is, they state that he/she will be able to: explain the purposes of the procedure, assemble the necessary equipment, prepare the patient emotionally and physically, assist with the insertion of the peritoneal catheter, monitor the patient during the procedure, and so on. The learning objective also should include a criterion for acceptable performance, and the conditions under which the behavior is to occur. This would include restrictions and limitations such as time; for example, within one week after beginning of instruction.

During the assessment or diagnostic phase of the teaching-process the nurse-manager works to determine what each subordinate knows or needs to know about the performance of a task. The nurse-manager may ask questions as subordinates perform a procedure under his/her direction, or the nurse-manager may demonstrate the procedure and invite the learners to ask questions or jot down points that need clarification later. If the nurse-manager is not knowledgeable about a task, he/she can use other resources that contribute to learning. Many nursing tasks are highly structured, having step-by-step details clearly delineated in a procedure manual or other written source. Others may not be so highly structured, requiring role modeling, discussion, or other methods for teaching.

planning

This is a shared responsibility so that everyone involved in the process helps decide how learning needs can be met. The planning phase provides a prescription for meeting learning needs. It should include a variety of techniques, both of teaching and learning. A nurse who is limited to one or two nursing activities is seriously handicapped in meeting the nursing needs of the patient. The same is true in teaching. The more learning activities and teaching techniques one has to choose from, the more individualized and effective the learning can be.

When planning how, when, and where learning will take place, it is well to keep in mind what research studies tell us about how people learn. According to authorities, people remember:

- 10% of what they read;
- 20% of what they hear;
- 30% of what they see;
- 50% of what they see and hear at the same time;
- 80% of what they say;
- 90% of what they say while doing a thing.

Teaching-learning techniques should be compatible with the desired behavioral objectives. One could spend endless hours lecturing on the topic of the use of monitoring equipment for cardiac patients and still not adequately describe the equipment and prepare someone to use it properly. A more appropriate technique would be to show the learner a diagram of the monitor and explain its use. But the most appropriate teaching-learning activities would include demonstrating use of the machine itself and giving learners practical experience in setting it up, attaching it to a person, and explaining to the instructor what they are doing at each step and why. Figure 6.4 gives an overview of appropriate techniques for different types of learning objectives.

The Department of Staff Development in most hospitals and clinics has access to a variety of audiovisual aids that can be made available to the nurse-manager. Various departments within the hospital or clinic as well as outside agencies also have resource persons and materials that can be useful in providing a variety of learning experiences for employees. When planning for the use of resource persons outside the patient care unit, the staff member inviting the person should be prepared to give specific information about his/her expectations for what the group hopes will be accomplished by the visit. It is unfair to invite someone in to talk about a subject without giving him/her some information about the people who will be in the audience. The resource person needs to know what the learners perceive to be their most pressing needs and objectives.

For example, if someone is invited to conduct a discussion on the topic of "helping the grieving family," that person should know if a general discussion of the grieving process is expected or if a more specific discussion is preferred. Do the members of the group need help in dealing with the spouses and children of adult patients with terminal cancer, or with the parents of children who are patients in an intensive care pediatric unit? The resource person can be much more effective if he/she knows the specific learning objectives of the group and how they think this person can be of help to them in achieving their objectives.

Besides the who, when, and where of teaching and learning one must, of course, consider the "what," that is, the content or subject matter to be covered. People vary in their capacity to learn as well as their inclination to do so. While the teacher must avoid assuming that some learners are either too dumb or too lazy to improve their level of performance, he/she also must be careful not to go to the other extreme and assume that everyone should and can learn the same amount of material and at the same pace.

Learning objectives are the structural framework of the content or subject matter. They should represent short steps toward accomplishment of a broader, more general goal. They should be sequenced in a logical order, so that progression is from the simple to the more difficult, from what is already known to what is yet to be learned. If they are individualized for each employee or level of nursing, then they will not be the same for a nurse attendant as they would be for an experienced professional nurse. Critical information or the "needs to know" for performance of a task should be clearly stated for each learner.

A good guideline to follow when planning instruction is to begin by finding out who needs to know what, and then determining who already has this critical knowledge. It may be that among the employees themselves there is a person who is knowledgeable and experienced enough in the area of content to serve as teacher for the group.

instruction

At this point much of the hard work has been done. Objectives have been determined, learning needs identified and individualized, and resources tapped to help meet those needs. Now should come the fun part.

Learning is a happy and ego-enhancing activity when it is seen as an opportunity to satisfy a yearning or fill a basic human need.

In a sense, learning is meeting the terms of a contract established between the teacher and the learner. In fact, in some schools students sign a contract stating exactly what they will do to earn a certain grade. In the less formal setting in which the nurse-manager operates, the contractual agreement might not be written, but it is there just the same. During the first two phases commitments have been made and witnessed by the members of the group. The objectives represent goals that presumably were considered important and achievable by the group. As plans were made, individuals accepted responsibility for doing their share in finding resource persons and materials, and being prepared for each session. In essence, the expectations each has for the others are the terms of a contract.

Studies have shown that "good" teachers are those who can be flexible. And flexibility can certainly be the saving grace of any nurse-manager who is assuming the role of teacher. No matter how carefully a learning activity might have been planned, there is always the possibility that something will happen to disrupt the planned activity. As long as the objectives are clear to everyone and opportunities to learn are present, changes in plans need not adversely affect the eventual outcome.

Much of the teaching taking place in a patient care unit can be spontaneous, on-the-spot, strike-while-the-iron-is-hot, kind of training. This is *not* to say that the first phases of the process are unnecessary; quite the contrary. Knowing the learning needs of employees and being prepared to meet those needs when the opportunity presents itself allow the nurse-manager to use spontaneity to advantage.

evaluation

It is during this phase that one determines whether the objectives have been achieved and learning needs met. Achievement of the objectives should result in a higher level of performance, more effective nursing care, increased confidence in employees and their ability to accept responsibility, and, quite possibly, a lower turnover rate among employees.

At the time evaluation is being done, every facet of the teaching-learning process should be reviewed one last time. If all objectives for the training period were not met, it may be that some were unrealistic in terms of the time and resources available and the ability of the employees to benefit from them. Or, the objectives could have been poorly constructed, too general, or not relevant to the situation in which they were to be used. This latter problem frequently occurs when objectives are borrowed from another source and not reviewed and revised so that they are better suited to the learners' individual needs. Another possibility is that the objectives were not sequenced in a logical and orderly progression, causing confusion in the learner. Or they might have covered more than small, "bite-sized" amounts of material. Objectives that make quantum leaps through large amounts of subject matter usually leave the learner floundering somewhere near the beginning of the instruction phase of the process.

Planned activities also should be appraised for their effectiveness in helping the learner to learn. Who, other than the learner, is better able to judge which techniques and resources were most helpful and which were not? The implication is that evaluation should be done by everyone involved in the process. The nurse-manager's main concern should be to what extent and in what specific areas did the training raise the level of competence of staff members and in what areas are they most likely to need further instruction. Answers to these and other questions could be most helpful in establishing new objectives and beginning the process all over again.

REFERENCES

[1] K. Davis, *Human Relations at Work*, 3rd ed., (New York: McGraw-Hill Book Co., 1967).

[2] J. A. S. Brown, *The Social Psychology of Industry*, (Baltimore: Penguin Books, Inc., 1954).

[3] E. Ghiselli, Managerial talent, *American Psychologist*, (Vol. 18, No. 10, 1963).

[4] C. L. Shartle, *Executive Performance and Leadership*, (Englewood Cliffs: Prentice-Hall, 1956).

[5] E. A. Fleishman and D. R. Peters, "Interpersonal values, leadership attitudes and managerial success," *Personnel Psychology*, (Vol. 15, 1962).

[6] R. Blake and J. Mouton, *Managerial Grid,* (Houston: Gulf Publishing, 1964).

[7] P. Hersey and K. Blanchard, *Management of Organizational Behavior*, (New Jersey: Prentice Hall, Inc., 1977).

[8] F. Fiedler, *A Theory of Leadership Effectiveness*, (New York: McGraw-Hill Book Co., 1967).

[9] *Ibid.*

[10]D. Votaw, "What do we believe about power?" reprinted from *California Management Review*, Vol. VIII, No. 4, in *Nursing Dimensions*, (Summer, 1979).

[11]H. Yurah and M. Walsh, "Concepts and theories related to leadership," *Nursing Dimensions*, (Summer, 1979).

[12]R. P. French and B. Raven, "The bases of social power," in *Studies in Social Power*, Dorwin Cartwright (ed.), (Ann Arbor: U. of Michigan, Institute for Social Research, 1959).

[13]R. B. Fine, "Applications of leadership theory: integrating thought and action," *Nursing Clinics of North America*, (March, 1978).

[14]F. Fiedler, *op. cit.*

[15]P. Hersey and K. Blanchard, *op. cit.*

[16]M. S. Knowles, *The Modern Practice of Adult Education*, (New York: Association Press, 1970).

SUGGESTED READINGS

J. A. Ashley, "Power, freedom and professional practice in nursing," *Supervisor Nurse*, (Jan., 1975).

C. Belanger, "Do you confront the boss?," *Supervisor Nurse*, (Dec., 1978).

M. Beyers and C. Phillips, "Keys to successful leadership," *Nursing 74 Book Section*, (July, 1974).

Sr. S. Courtade, "The role of the head nurse: Power and practice," *Supervisor Nurse*, (Dec., 1978).

R. B. Fine, "Applications of leadership theory: Integrating thought and action," *Nursing Clinics of North America*, (March, 1978).

C. G. Heimann, "Four theories of leadership," *Journal of Nursing Administration*, (June, 1976).

P. Hersey et al., "A situational approach to supervision: Leadership theory and the supervising nurse," *Supervisor Nurse*, (May, 1976).

P. Hersey et al., "A look at your supervisory style," *Supervisor Nurse*, (June, 1976).

T. Kron, "How to become a better leader," *Nursing 76*, (Oct., 1976).

A. Levenstein, "Leading the troops," *Supervisor Nurse*, (March, 1975).

J. K. Mann, "Nursing leadership in the critical care setting," *Nursing Clinics of North America*, (March, 1978).

P. Nelson, "Instantaneous leadership," *Supervisor Nurse*, (March, 1975).

R. Pritchard, "A philosophy of reaching applied to administration," *Journal of Nursing Administration*, (Sept., 1975).

A. G. Sargent, "The androgynous manager," *Supervisor Nurse*, (March, 1979).

D. Votaw, "What do we believe about power?," *Nursing Dimensions*, (Summer, 1979).

H. Yurah and M. Walsh, "Concepts and theories related to leadership," *Nursing Dimensions*, (Summer, 1979).

chapter 7

index

chapter
communication

All living systems, whether human or organizational, depend on a communication network to receive and transmit messages so that the diverse functions of the system can be coordinated and integrated. The communication network of an organization is somewhat analogous to the nervous system of the human body. Messages picked up from the external and internal environments are transmitted throughout the body where they elicit various kinds of responses. Physiologic problems develop when messages are not received, transmitted, or responded to appropriately.

In an organization, problems arise because it is falsely assumed that all messages sent by one element of the system are *received*, fully *understood* as intended by the sender, and *accepted* by the receivers. Decision making, communication, and action are all interrelated and interdependent functions of the individuals who work at various levels in an organization. If there is misunderstanding or rejection of the messages sent and received by these individuals, the communication network is rendered ineffective.

Researchers estimate that managers spend from 75 to 95 percent of their time communicating. As first-line manager you are involved in interpersonal communication with subordinates, peers, and superiors, and in organizational communication via formal and informal channels. In the process of communication you will be concerned with both the content of the messages and the emotional and attitudinal factors that influence acceptance or rejection of a message.

In this chapter we will discuss the nature of communication and the strategies and techniques you can use to overcome barriers to communication. Because effective listening is such an essential part of effective communication, we will discuss how you might employ some techniques of active listening to facilitate communication. Finally, the topic of delegation and its relationship to communication skills is briefly explored and some suggestions are offered to help you delegate tasks and responsibilities more successfully.

THE NATURE OF COMMUNICATION

Communication can be defined in its simplest form as the flow of messages.[1] *Effective* communication is an exchange of meanings between and among individuals through a *shared* system of symbols. That is, both sender and receiver of the message must know what the symbols mean to one another if the message is to be acted upon appropriately. Verbal communication depends on the transmission of mutually understood words. Nonverbal communication, which psychologists believe speaks much more powerfully than verbal communication, includes facial expressions, eye contact, touch and body movements, rate of speech, tone of voice, and inflections.

Verbal and nonverbal communications transmit *concepts* (cognitive material) and *feelings* (motivational and emotional material).[2] Examples of *cognitive material* that is transmitted in an organization include information or facts about the tasks performed; ideas, suggestions, and experiences of the individuals; and knowledge of policies, actions, and objectives of individuals and the organization. These are the kinds of message materials that we most often think of when we consider the content of communication. Managers most certainly must consider the clarity of content when they prepare messages for transmission. Later we will discuss this aspect of communication and the responsibilities of the sender as well as those of the receiver during the transmission of ideas.

Examples of *motivational and emotional material,* as described by Likert, include the emotional environment or atmosphere through which the message travels; the attitudes and personal reactions of senders and receivers; their loyalties, hostilities, feelings of support and rejection; and their personal goals and objectives. The effective exchange of ideas must take place in an environment that permits clear transmission of the message. Environmental "noise" produced by emotions distorts messages in the same way that disturbances in the atmosphere surrounding the earth can create static on a radio or distortion of a television picture.

Unfavorable attitudes and incompatible goals and objectives, whether implicitly or explicitly stated by the receiver, can create serious barriers to the flow of messages. If, for example, you delegate responsibility for the performance of a task to a subordinate and the subordinate perceives the task as unimportant, an imposition, unreasonable, or incompatible with his/her objectives, your continued efforts to clarify the cognitive ingredients of the message will not guarantee acceptance of your message and compliance with your wishes.

An example of the way in which emotional responses can prevent effective communication is an incident that occurred during a class session which, incidentally, was on the topic of communication. Two participants were involved in what was supposed to be an exchange of ideas relevant to a problem that was of great importance to one of them but of only passing interest to the other. They started out calmly enough, but in a short while their voices rose, they became openly hostile toward one another, and were speaking almost simultaneously. It was painfully obvious that neither was listening to the other, and certainly neither was communicating anything more than raw emotion. Finally, one of them said, "You just don't understand what I'm saying!" To which the other replied, "You're not saying anything that can be understood!" At this point the entire class broke into laughter, including the two who were having their troubles communicating. The tension was relieved and the climate changed to one in which there was more acceptance and therefore better reception of the message.

The example points out some of the factors that can either enhance or impede the flow of messages. A more comprehensive definition must take into account the purpose for which the message is being sent and whether the response of the sender indicates that the desired effect has been achieved. Effective communication is a concern of every manager. Communication that is effective is that in which the sending and receiving of ideas, feelings, and attitudes results in a favorable response.[3] Both the stimulus and the response in communication arises from verbal and nonverbal behavior of the people involved. Of the two, nonverbal behavior most often expresses the *true social meaning* of a message sent during a face-to-face communication.[4]

MODELS OF COMMUNICATION

A communication system can be *intrapersonal*, as for example, when you think and talk to yourself; *interpersonal*, in which case the flow of messages is between two or more persons; and *intraorganizational*, that is, the transmission of messages along formal and informal channels within the organization. In each kind of communication, the purpose is *understanding*. In an organizational system the ultimate purpose of communication is achieving some level of understanding and agreement about decisions that are being made, communicating the content and purpose of mutually-agreed-upon decisions, and converting them into activities that help meet the goals of the organization.

There are three critical elements in a model depicting the structure and process of intrapersonal, interpersonal, and intraorganizational communication. These are the sender, the message, and the receiver. The source of the message is within the sender, who produces an original idea or borrows one from another source for the purpose of transmitting to it. Once the idea is formulated, however incompletely or imperfectly, the sender must *encode* it. Encoding requires converting the idea into some kind of verbal or nonverbal symbol or set of symbols that is intended to have meaning to the receiver. This encoded message is then sent via a formal or informal channel to the receiver.

The message is then received and *decoded* by the receiver. By decoding is meant the reconstruction of the idea according to the receiver's ability to understand the message. Understanding is improved if there is time and a means is provided for feedback and verification. As we have said, barriers to communication can prevent a smooth flowing of messages. Since communication does not take place in a sterile and nonviable environment, the entire process must be considered in the context in which the communication is taking place. Figure 7.1 shows a model of communication in which each of these components and elements are considered.

A common problem of communication that produces an inappropriate response is that of a disparity between the meaning *intended* by the sender and the meaning that is accepted and acted upon by the receiver. Sometimes the results can be disastrous, as in the case of administering the wrong drug or treatment to a patient, and sometimes the outcome is ludicrous.

figure 7.1   model of communication

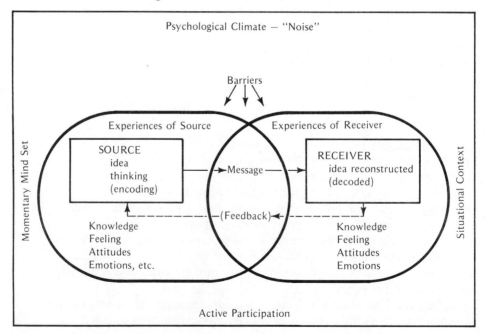

A rather humorous example is one that occurred when a visiting foreign dignitary was being welcomed to a small town in Tennessee. The state flower is the iris, which is also known locally as a "flag." When the dignitary arrived he was greeted by the school children of the town, who were lined up along the main street waving American flags. All of the children, that is, except one group who were standing in the blazing sun holding wilted state flowers. Their teacher had been told to have each of her students bring a flag to the celebration and wave it upon entry of the dignitary. The teacher heard "flag" and decoded it to "iris." Such a translation seemed perfectly sensible to her and appropriate for the occasion. No harm was done and, once they overcame their embarrassment, the children were able to laugh about it.

But not all breakdowns in communication have such happy endings nor are they always the result of erroneous translation of words. Even when the factual parts of a communication are properly encoded, the implications for the receiver can be misunderstood because of the receiver's needs, motives, and past experiences. This is true whether we are talking about interpersonal communication, as between a head nurse and one or more of her employees, or organizational communication, which is a more formal system for transmission of information and meaning to large numbers of people within an agency.

For our purposes here we will limit discussion of communication to interpersonal exchanges of ideas and messages. The same principles apply to all types of communication, but as a first-line manager you are primarily responsible for sending and receiving messages to and from your subordinates, co-workers, and immediate supervisors.

THE COMMUNICATION PROCESS

It is difficult to analyze communication and separate its components into neat compartments because it is a process during which numerous things are operating simultaneously. So many things, in fact, that we can only look at it analytically as one might view a single frame of a moving picture. We stop the projector, look at the picture, and try to describe what is happening at that given moment. Such a view does not reveal the full dynamics of communication, but it does help us to see the basic elements of the process. We will begin our analysis by discussing the source of the message.

conceiving the message

As we have said, a message begins as an idea within the mind of the sender. It can be an original idea or one that is borrowed from another source. In any case, once the decision is made to share the idea with someone else, it is the origin of the message that eventually will be transmitted. If at all possible, the integrity of the idea should be maintained throughout the process so that it arrives at its destination and is understood as intended by the sender.

credibility

Whether or not the source can be believed and trusted is a major factor in the receiver's acceptance of the message. The source could be a piece of writing, a person, or a group. If the source is considered to be truthful, reliable, and trustworthy, the message has a much better chance of getting through to and favorably influencing the receiver. For example, a source that should have a high credibility rating is a well-established nursing journal. One that would not have much credibility as a source of scientific information for the practice of nursing might be a periodical such as those we see at the checkout counter in the supermarket.

Sometimes head nurses and team leaders unwittingly destroy the credibility of a source by saying something such as, "I am not sure who said you should take only 30 minutes for lunch, but I think it was . . . ." A perfectly natural response to this kind of message is to ignore it until something a little more authoritative is communicated.

Your expert power is related to your own credibility as the source of a message. If you know what you are talking about when you write a nursing order, and your subordinates have faith in your nursing judgment, the messages that you transmit to them have a better chance of being understood and accepted as you intended. This is particularly true when you are delegating nursing duties and responsibilities.

Lack of credibility obstructs a listener's ability to hear what is being said and a reader's ability to read and understand what has been written. A credibility gap between the source and the receiver contributes to environmental noise that distorts the message. If the source is not trusted by the receiver, the message may be rejected completely. The receiver is "turned off" by the source and does not want to accept the message.

You can increase your own credibility as a source by double checking the sources that *you* use. It is important that you know the author and publisher of printed material, and by all means check the date of publication. A hospital procedure book might seem to be a good bet as a reliable source and it usually is, unless it was written in the 1960's and hasn't been revised since.

If it is your responsibility to pass messages from higher levels of management to your employees, be very sure that you know their origin and understand what is intended in each message. Find out who wrote the message and seek an opportunity to give feedback so that you can ask questions and clarify in your own mind what it says. If you don't do this, you may find yourself saying to your subordinates, "Well, I'm not sure what it means. Maybe you should ask the supervisor." Once you have done this, you have lost some of your own credibility and authoritative power.

Credibility has as much to do with *how* you say something as *what* you say. Frequently you will need to persuade your subordinates to take a message seriously and act on it in an appropriate manner. Research studies have shown that you can be more persuasive if you: (1) appear to know what you are talking about; (2) believe in what you are saying; and (3) behave in a convincing way. This brings us to the subject of assertiveness and the effect the behavior of the sender has on the message and how it is received during the communication process.

assertiveness and communication

You convey all kinds of messages through your actions and tone of voice as well as what you say when communicating with someone else. You can very submissively say, "I really do need you to help serve the breakfast trays each morning if you aren't too busy." Or you can be aggressive and say through clenched teeth in a loud voice, "You just keep finding something else to do every time the breakfast trays need to be served and you'll be finding another job!" Or, you can speak calmly and assertively and say, "I know you are quite busy in the mornings, but I want you to help serve breakfast trays so the patients can get them while the food is hot."

Assertiveness has been touted as the miracle cure for the ills of modern women. It isn't any such thing, of course, but the skills and techniques learned during assertiveness training most assuredly are helpful in getting a message across and accomplishing goals that are important to you.

The best way to learn these techniques and develop your skill in being assertive is by actively learning and practicing them. Usually this is done in a workshop setting in which the learners can take part in role playing, demonstrations, discussions, and other learning activities involving participation and interaction with other people. Assertiveness is not easily learned just by reading about it. Sooner or later you are going to have to try your skill in dealing with someone else. If you want to be more assertive than you are and have not had an opportunity to attend an assertiveness program, you ought to do so as soon as you can. In the meantime, an overview of what it is all about can help you decide whether you already have the skills needed or could use some help in learning how to communicate your thoughts clearly when in emotionally threatening situations.

First of all assertiveness is a set of *learned attitudes* and *communication skills* that can be changed so that feelings of uneasiness and personal inadequacy can be overcome.[5] Assertiveness is defined by Baer as "making your own choices, standing up for yourself appropriately, and having an active orientation to life." Standing up for your rights does not mean that the rights of others must be violated.[6] Assertiveness is neither passiveness nor aggressiveness, but rather a way of acting that improves your self-esteem and helps you communicate clearly and firmly your objectives and personal needs.

The goal of assertiveness training is to make you feel better about yourself without aggressively putting down other people. It is based on the belief that a change in your behavior will gradually bring about a change in your attitudes about yourself. The training provides specific skills and techniques to help you get control of yourself and be less shy or less aggressive and hostile. Some of us lack these skills, and because of past experiences in our dealings with others we vacillate between being too submissive and or aggressive. We are unable to accept compliments; unable to say "no" when we want to say "no" and do it without feeling guilty; unable to say "yes" when we want to say "yes;" and unable to speak up whenever we feel justified in doing so. Assertiveness training is designed to help overcome these barriers so that a person can express himself or herself and communicate wants and feelings.

Throughout the rest of this chapter we will be talking about techniques for effective communication. Many of these, including nonverbal as well as verbal behavior, are a part of assertiveness. They include facing the person with whom you are talking and establishing eye contact, using appropriate gestures and facial expressions to increase the impact of your words, and choosing simple and direct language to say exactly what you think, feel, and want.

encoding the message

Most of us think we learned to communicate when we learned to talk, read, and write. But these are only the ingredients that we have to work with. It is something like baking a cake from scratch. The end product of our efforts at communicating and the end product of the baking process can be either satisfying or sadly disappointing, depending on how we put it together.

It would not occur to us probably to blame the people who sampled our cake if they failed to enjoy it. Yet often that is what we do when a message that we have concocted fails to convey to its recipient what we intended when we encoded it. The point is that the sender must bear responsibility for preparing and sending a message so that it can be decoded by the receiver with minimal difficulty.

There will be times when you will need to decide whether it would be best to communicate orally, in writing, or both. Most of the time you will communicate with your subordinates orally, giving directions, asking and answering questions, settling disputes, and handling minor conflicts. These usually are appropriate occasions for oral communication.[7]

At other times a written communication is most effective. These would include a need to communicate information that requires employee action in the *future*. Patient care assignments, nursing orders, and exceptions to routine care are better as written, rather than oral directives, which can be forgotten or misunderstood or both.

Sometimes it is best to use oral communication and then follow up with a written message. This is true when the information being communicated demands immediate action on the part of employees, as when there is an agency directive or order that directly affects their work. The commendation of an employee for work well done should be both oral and written. If you keep a copy of the commendation, it will come in handy when evaluation time rolls around. Information about a problem that requires the help of a supervisor or other higher level manager should be communicated orally followed by a written report.[8]

oral messages

When you are giving directions, providing information, and asking questions verbally, there is a very good chance that you will be misunderstood if you don't follow the rules of good communication. Some of these rules are:

1. *Speak slowly and distinctly.* Slowing down gives you time to organize your thoughts a little better and helps the receiver decode more easily. Our brains operate at a higher speed than our tongues, so we often leave out words we thought we had said when we are talking rapidly. A slower pace lets you finish sentences, something you might not do if you are trying to verbalize every thought as soon as it comes into your head. Try listening to every word spoken by someone who is talking at a rapid-fire pace. You probably will hear half-finished thoughts and incomplete sentences.

2. *Pause between every sentence or two and let the words "sink in."* You need to listen to what *you* are saying and take time to correct any errors that may have crept into your message. During the pauses look for feedback such as facial expressions, body gestures, and other signals that tell you whether or not you are being understood.

3. *Avoid giving more than one or two verbal directives at one time.* If there are more than that, you had better write them down for the receiver. Don't expect an employee to remember and carry out a laundry list of "things I want you to do today." There will be many distractions during the day and the employee probably won't remember half of what you have said. Chances are that you yourself will not be able to recall everything either.

4. *Use redundancy in your message.* Experts tell us that repetition of the basic elements of a message is the greatest enemy of the audio and visual static that can damage the integrity of the message. Fortunately, most written and spoken messages transmitted at any given time are about half redundant anyway. If 50 percent of the words in a written paragraph or radio broadcast were deleted, the message probably would be understood. That is, the central theme would be received, but some of the details probably would be lost. As you are well aware, it is the loss of these "little details" that causes drug errors, mistaken identity of patients, and similar incidents that bring about premature aging in nurse-managers. That is why you are urged to check to be sure you have repeated the important points when encoding and transmitting a verbal communication to your employees and co-workers.

5. *Ask for feedback.* If an employee cannot repeat what you have said in her own words, and accurately give back the details, your message has not been received as intended. The employee might be insulted by your asking for feedback, but that should not bother you. If the message is important enough for you to communicate to an employee, it is important enough for her to try to understand. Be assertive, and just say you want her to tell you whether she understands and if so, exactly what she understood your message to say.

6. *Face the person you are speaking to and establish eye contact.* This tells the person that your message is important and that you want his/her attention while you are speaking. It also tells the receiver that he/she is a vital part of the communication process and you are willing to take the time needed to deliver a message and be sure it is received. Looking down or letting your eyes rest on something other than the receiver is submissive, nonassertive behavior. When you are giving an order or supplying needed information to an employee you must talk and act as if you mean what you are saying.

written messages

Nurse managers are expected to submit written reports upward to supervisors and administrators, laterally to colleagues and co-workers, and downward to employees. The rules for written communication are equally important, no matter in which direction the message is to be transmitted. Here are some suggestions for improving your written communications:

1. *Keep it simple and direct.* Use short words and short sentences. In recent times some unhappy citizens have formed an organization to combat the unintelligible reports and directions issued by various offices of the federal government. But unreadable messages are not

limited to government reports. Many memos from personnel departments, administrative offices, and other levels of management are difficult to understand because it isn't easy to reduce complex messages into simple language. We all are tempted to use big words in writing; otherwise we think our intelligence and creativity will be questioned. The truth is that while fancy language and long sentences may indicate an extensive vocabulary and knowledge of the rules of punctuation, they create environmental noise that interferes with effective communication.

If you want to get an idea of the grade level at which something has been written, whether by you or someone else, there are several formulas for determining this. The most popular formula was developed by Robert Gunning. It is not the most accurate, but it is the simplest to use and does give a quick way to estimate how easy or difficult it is to read any piece of writing. The Gunning formula is:

Reading grade level = 0.4 (average sentence length + percentage of words of three or more syllables).

- Count 100-word sample (or to end of sentence).
- Count number of sentences.
- Compute average sentence length by dividing number of words in sample by number of sentences.
- Count number of words having three syllables or more, with these exceptions: omit compound words or words that form their third syllable by adding es, ed, ly, ing, etc.
- Compute formula.
- A number of samples should be used and averaged. The higher the reading level, the more difficult it is to understand the meaning of the message.

2. *Encode beforehand.* Remember that ideas are not born fully developed. Jot down what you think you want to say, let it sit for a while, think about it, and then go back and read what you have written. Does it really say what you want it to? Have you said too much or too little? Is it written in a logical and organized manner or are central ideas scattered throughout in a haphazard way?

Try to read it as if someone else had written the words. Then try to read it from the viewpoint of the people you are hoping to communicate with. A good rule of thumb for checking to be sure you have included the most important parts of the message is to go over the five W's: Who, what, when, where, and why. If it is important to state *how* a directive is to be carried out, then that must also be included.

3. *Organize written messages.* If you have encoded properly beforehand, it should be relatively easy to look at what you have written and then

organize it so that the main message will get across intact. Your most important point should be stated first, then the next most important, and so on. Edit your writing, deleting unnecessary words and ideas that could distract the reader from the central message. Substitute short words for long ones wherever possible. Rewrite long sentences so that they are broken down into short and to-the-point statements.

4. *Encode messages in words that are meaningful to the receiver.* Words have different meanings to people. Redundancy can help eliminate error and so can using measurable terms when you want to indicate an amount. For example, "Repeated instances of tardiness will require make-up time or an adjustment in pay" is not nearly so clear and easily understood as, "If you are late for work more than two times during any pay period, you must make up the time or take a cut in pay for the time you were not at work."

Encoding a message properly so as to avoid misunderstanding requires time. It forces you to think through what you want to say before transmitting the words to someone else. Write it as you would say it, then look at the message and ask, "How could it possibly be misunderstood?"

5. *Be neat.* The appearance of a written message adds or detracts from its meaning and impact. A note hastily scratched on the back of a scrap of used paper speaks volumes about the attitude of the sender. And woe to you who use history sheets, nurse's notes, and other expensive printed forms to jot down a note to an employee or colleague. You can't talk about being orderly and frugal and then write a sloppy and disorganized note on a piece of stationary that was printed for some other purpose. Whoever sees and reads the message is going to have more than the meanings of the words communicated to her.

BARRIERS AND FACILITATORS IN COMMUNICATION

It has been said that communication is like the weather; everybody talks about it, but nobody seems to be able to do much about it. Weather and communication do pervade every aspect of our lives, and they both have the potential for making us joyful or miserable. The best we can do is create our own environment in which the harmful effects are minimized and the benefits maximized.

Communication is a dynamic process taking place in a complex and active environment. Little wonder that so many things can go wrong and often do. Even more wonderful is the fact that in spite of the hazards, we all manage to communicate to some degree even though communication rarely is perfect. We can do this because of our ability to "speak" in so many different ways, overcoming many of the barriers that impede the transmission of messages. These barriers include external and internal factors capable of distorting and sometimes even blocking completely the flow of meaning.[9]

Among the external factors are sensory stimuli at distract the receiver and prevent concentration on the meaning of the message. The internal factors include those psychological, cultural and social stimuli that cloud the perception of the receiver and cause misunderstanding or outright rejection of the intended meaning. If you have ever wondered how on earth a subordinate, peer, or supervisor could have misunderstood a message that was so clearly stated and perfectly encoded, it may very well be that the environment through which the message was sent distorted your meaning. Or it may be that the receiver was not psychologically or emotionally able to accept your intended meaning because it was not comparable with his/her values and attitudes.

external factors

Some of the most obvious barriers to effective communication are the physical circumstances in which a message is sent. Experts call these sets of circumstances "noise," but they are talking about more than auditory interference.

Besides the sound of ringing phones, distracting conversations held nearby, and other environmental sounds, there are physical barriers such as desks, plate glass windows, and half-opened or completely closed doors. One of the cardinal rules for encoding and transmitting messages is to try to develop empathy for the receiver. This is not as easy as it sounds. For the next few days, when you are in the role of receiver of messages and are having difficulty understanding their meaning, stop and survey your immediate environment. What sights, sounds, and perhaps even smells, are getting in your way?

In order to overcome some of these barriers we must first become aware of their influence on effective communication, and then we can take steps to avoid them. Experts tell us that a good way to do this is by *isolating the message*; that is, removing it from disruptive factors insofar as is possible. For example, a written message that you want your employees to read should be put in a spot where it does not have to compete with a lot of other written messages. A note to employees telling them about an in-service education program that they are required to attend probably won't be read if it is tacked to a bulletin board cluttered with memos, outdated material, and other less urgent messages.

If your message is to be delivered verbally, take the person or persons receiving it to a quiet place where they will be free from interruption and distractions. You don't need to make a big production of it. Just take the receiver aside, away from the environmental noise, deliver your message, and seek input to be sure your intended meaning has been conveyed and accepted.

If it is not possible to isolate the message, then efforts at obtaining immediate feedback should be doubled so that any misunderstandings can be cleared up and details repeated as necessary. When you ask for and receive responses from the receiver and then repeat the message in a different way, you are providing opportunities for overcoming environmental noise.

Another noise factor might be the *pressure of time*. When either the sender or the receiver is rushed, it is difficult to concentrate on what is being said verbally or in writing. Attention is diverted to whatever must be done next, rather than what is being said and done *now*. It takes self-discipline to get control of yourself and focus your thoughts on the task of communicating. Once you are able to do this and demand the same kind of attention from your employees, the fewer mistakes they will make when carrying out duties you have delegated to them.

Much of the communicating that you do as a first-line manager is verbal. While it is quicker and easier to speak messages than to write them, it is not always the most efficient channel to use in the long run. Many people are poor listeners, and they are even less likely to be attentive when they are working under pressure.

In the previous chapter we noted that people remember less than one-fourth of what they have heard. If you are having problems with your employees carrying out your verbal directives, it may very well be that you have chosen the wrong channel for communicating with them. Or, you might have chosen the wrong path. The more people involved in a chain of communication, the more likely it is that the message will be misunderstood by the person for whom it was intended ultimately.

Remember the game of "gossip"? The original statement is so distorted by the time it reaches the last person in line it is not recognizable. The moral here is that people unwittingly mistranslate words that they hear, filter out those they don't want to hear, and thus lose the intended meaning of the message. If you want to minimize the risk of losing the meaning during translation, write down exactly what you mean and then deliver the message directly to the ultimate receiver. A more hazardous path is to give the *written* message to someone else for delivery. The most hazardous route is that of a *verbal* message delivered through one or more persons before it reaches its final destination.

internal factors

Even though it is not always easy to identify external barriers to communication, it certainly is less difficult than trying to understand what is going on in the minds and emotions of the receivers of messages. All manner of problems can develop because the person either does not have the intellectual capacity to understand or is emotionally unable to accept the meaning.

If the intellectual capacity of the receiver is such that he/she cannot understand what you are saying, then "watch your language" and use simple words. If the message is complex, break it down into short steps and deliver them one at a time, asking for feedback and clarifying your meaning at the end of each step. This could be an opportunity for diagnosing the learning needs of your subordinates. You might find that some of them are not following through on tasks delegated to them because they do not understand what is to be done and how to do it.

Emotional reactions that can create barriers to communication arise from any of a number of reasons.

lack of interest on the part of the receiver. A perfectly natural question in the mind of every receiver is, "What's in it for me?" This is an automatic response whenever someone tries to get our attention and hold it throughout the transmission of a message. When you are encoding a message, look for valid reasons why the receiver should be interested in what you are saying, and present these reasons before giving the message.

value differences. There are topics of communication which are positively valued by some persons and negatively valued by others. You might feel that the spiritual aspects of patient care are of great importance in promoting healing, but when you try to communicate your concern and provide information on the subject to some of your subordinates, you find they are "turned off by religion" and unable to accept your message. On the other hand, they may be very excited about new policies related to formation of a union and increase in pay, while you have very negative feelings about this.

Differences in values need not create an insurmountable obstacle to communication. As long as you are sensitive to the possibility that such differences could exist, and are willing to work around them if at all possible, you may be able to communicate more effectively with your employees in spite of differing values.

lack of trust in the sender. People transfer their feelings about the sender of a message to the message itself. If the receivers are confident that the sender is honest, knowledgeable, and a person of integrity, they will accept the message. If not, they will reject the message, refusing to believe what is said. We have already discussed this barrier to communication when we talked about credibility of the sender.

The only way you can overcome this barrier is to develop a sense of mutual trust between yourself and the receiver. Once credibility is lost it is difficult, if not impossible, to regain. Above all, be honest and never forget that actions do indeed speak louder than words. If your actions contradict your words, you will be judged either as a manipulator of people or as a person who lacks integrity. In a book titled *Is Anybody Listening?* W. H.

Whyte wrote: "Only with trust can there be any real communication, and until that trust is achieved, the gadgetry of communications are so much wasted effort."

conflict with lifetime habits. Credibility and trust in the sender do not automatically guarantee acceptance of the message and compliance with its directives. If the content of a communication is not in accord with well-entrenched habitual behavior, the message can be accepted as factual and yet ignored completely.

This can be a very real problem for the first-line manager who wants to institute some change in the work activities of employees in her department. She can present some very good reasons why, for example, a team leader should accept more responsibility for evaluating and upgrading the performance of her team members. But if the team leader is not comfortable in a position of authority and has habitually acted like "one of the girls" when dealing with her team members, she will ignore the message and continue to function as she has in the past. This usually is not a deliberate, premeditated act of insubordination. The team leader might not even be aware that she has failed to hear and accept the message.

The task of the nurse-manager faced with this kind of communication problem is to bring it out into the open and have an honest dialogue with the person who is having difficulty receiving her messages. Rather than blame the employee for laziness or lack of initiative, it is better to look for reasons why she is not motivated to accept more responsibility. If she can be convinced that changing her ways of behaving is to her own advantage there is a much better chance that she will respond favorably to communications calling for a change in her behavior. Until she is motivated to react positively, written and verbal messages will be ignored and her old way of doing things will prevail.

status and power differences. In ancient times it was the custom to reward the bearer of good news and execute the bearer of bad news. There remains to this day a vestige of fear that we will be blamed personally for communicating an unpleasant message. The result is a kind of noncommunication, in which information is withheld for fear of reprisal. In the area of management, subordinates withhold important information from their supervisors if they think that such information might in some way be a reflection on their competence. As a first-line manager you may have difficulty communicating upward because of a reluctance to pass on some unpleasant news. You might think that telling your supervisor about a problem you are having would indicate your inability to deal with something that you should be able to resolve. And you may not receive information from your subordinates for the same reason.

Communication also can be impeded between persons having different levels of power and influence because the person of lesser power is awed by the other person's position of authority, real or imagined. The message becomes obscured by emotions arising from an acute awareness of the status difference. You might have difficulty communicating with a leader in nursing whom you have admired from a distance for years and now have occasion to chat with informally. On the other hand, you yourself may have difficulty getting a message across to a new employee who is young and inexperienced and whose perspective of nursing is vastly different from yours. She may be in awe of your experience and expertise in nursing and your status as head nurse, and her emotions block out messages from you.

One way you can help overcome this barrier is to carry on communication in an environment in which the receiver is most at ease. If an employee is having difficulty hearing your messages because of emotional "noise," let her decide where she would like to talk with you. During your conversation be aware of the negative effects of physical barriers, for example, the desk between you, and remove them if possible. Avoid facial expressions, tone of voice, and other nonverbal language that is likely to increase her discomfort and make her more aware of your status as manager. Work toward developing her self-confidence by showing that you believe in her potential and her worth as a valued employee.

EFFECTIVE LISTENING

The other half of the communication process is that of receiving messages. Listening, *really* listening and concentrating on what you are hearing is not easy. The trouble is, most of us are talking out loud (or to ourselves) when we should be listening. We do this because we are impressed with our own wisdom and the importance of what we have to say (as soon as we get the chance), or because we are insecure and afraid to be open to ideas and suggestions that may be contrary to our own, or because we simply don't want to be bothered with hearing someone else's thoughts and opinions.

Carl R. Rogers, in his writing on breakdowns in communication, identifies three basic elements of effective listening. They are: (1) the development of a certain attitude; (2) the skilled control of a definite strategy; and (3) a set of techniques.[10]

attitudes

A prerequisite to being a good listener is the desire to hear and accept what the other person is saying. There must be a conviction that the messages being sent are important and worthy of the receiver's attention. And there should be a willingness to sit still and listen without interrupting or distracting the speaker.

It takes discipline and self-control to be quiet and relaxed when another person is speaking, especially if emotions are high, or if the speaker is rambling, inarticulate, or saying something we don't especially want to hear. Most of us have difficulty keeping our minds from wandering while someone else is speaking, and yet the art of effective listening is based on a willingness to devote our *whole attention* to the speaker and to actively help him or her communicate more effectively.

strategy

A strategy is a set of plans to accomplish a goal. When you are actively listening you are not just giving the speaker an opportunity to talk about whatever is on his/her mind or to vent emotions. That may well be part of your plan if your goal is to build confidence in the employee and permit her to talk about matters of importance to her, but you also will want to get some facts about a particular situation.

If you are talking with an employee about a specific problem, your goal should be to obtain information that will be helpful in identifying the problem and finding a solution. Perhaps the employee is not performing at an acceptable level and you want to know why. Or there may be interpersonal conflicts among staff members that are interfering with their work.

Another reason for actively listening to an employee might be to obtain information about the kind of nursing care that is being provided on your unit. Whatever your goal, you are the manager and you should remain in control of what is happening during an interview no matter how short or informal.

Let's say, for example, that a nurse attendant who has been a dependable and competent employee begins to leave her work unfinished and is often late for work. You arrange for her to come to your office to talk about the change in her behavior. When you ask what is troubling her she says, "I guess I'm just tired of nursing and need to do something else for a living."

At this point you can accept what she has said, ask for her resignation, and terminate the interview. Or you can use some listening techniques to get at the real reason why her performance level has become unsatisfactory. In either case, you should know what you are doing and why you have chosen a specific way to deal with the problem. Perhaps you agree that the nurse attendant should seek employment elsewhere, but if you are really interested in helping her regain her position as a valuable employee, you are going to have to do more than sit there like a lump and passively accept whatever she says. You're going to have to be assertive and creative to be helpful.

Sometimes it is the employee who initiates a discussion. You still need to be in control and to set some goals for the communication that will take place. Being in control means using techniques that will help you and the person you are communicating with have a meaningful and fruitful exchange of thought.

techniques

Psychologists and psychiatrists depend very heavily on the art of communication to practice their professions. It is from them that we have learned such helpful procedures as *nondirective counseling* and *nondirective interviewing*. This is not to suggest that as manager you take on the task of psychologic counseling, but rather that you use specific listening techniques in order to help your employees speak more freely and provide information that will help you and them get the job done.

The first of these techniques involves *setting the stage* so that the speaker and listener can get to the point of the discussion or interview as quickly as possible. Small talk and meaningless amenities about the weather, one's state of health, and so forth are a waste of time. They can produce anxiety and frustration for the employee who wants to get on with the interview and get back to work or go home.

The stage is set by making a short statement as to the topic to be discussed. It might be something like, "We need to talk about the problem you are having with your charting. What do you think the trouble might be?" As the employee talks, the manager listens patiently and resists the temptation to criticize, evaluate and make judgments, sermonize, or give advice.

Ruth Strebe suggests that when you first begin practicing your listening skills, you work at analyzing your own thoughts during an exchange. Ask yourself whether you are "thinking with" the speaker and trying to get a sense of the total meaning of the words and feelings in the message. Are you "thinking advice" as you listen and focusing on what she should do or feel rather than on what she is experiencing at the moment? Are you making judgments and reacting with your own point of view? And, finally, are you thinking about the content of the words and ignoring evidence of feelings that are also being transmitted?[11]

Active listening is hard work, requiring all your powers of concentration and an added dose of intuition. An active listener is involved. An active listener cares about the person as well as what he or she is communicating.

Two other techniques that help a speaker communicate effectively are called *reflective summary* and *probing*. After listening carefully to the speaker and receiving verbal and nonverbal messages, the listener makes an attempt to summarize the total sense of the message. This is not easy to do because there is a tendency to let emotions and values affect translation and to respond by using words and phrases that imply a criticism, good or bad, of what has been transmitted. If, for example, the gist of the message is that an employee feels that she is being assigned to perform tasks for which she has not been prepared by training or experience, you would repeat the message as you understand it. You might say, "You are saying that you have not been taught how to carry out some of the nursing procedures that have been assigned to you?'' The sender may then reply, ''Yes, and I don't think I should be expected to do some of them. After all, I just graduated a few months ago.'' Now, it seems, the employee has more on her mind than a feeling of inadequacy in the performance of certain nursing procedures.

At this point you can use the techniques of probing. This is done only after you have restated the ideas and feelings of the speaker accurately and to her satisfaction. The probing technique requires sensitivity to the feelings of the speaker. It is done for the purpose of helping her get across the thoughts that she is having difficulty expressing. It goes without saying that whatever is uncovered by probing is accepted uncritically and treated as confidential information unless the speaker wishes otherwise. There must be mutual trust and respect if probing is to elicit the information you need.

Van Dersal suggests that an active listener should keep three kinds of questions in mind while the speaker is talking.[12] First, ''What does the speaker mean?'' Try to translate the words as you think she intends and then ask such questions as, ''Do I understand you to mean . . . . If I understand you correctly, you are saying that . . . .''

The second group of questions should help you decide whether the speaker really knows what she is talking about. This doesn't mean that you challenge every statement, or that you doubt her veracity, but rather you want to deal with factual information insofar as it is possible to obtain it. After the speaker has finished talking, you should carefully and cautiously try to clarify, in both your mind and hers, what has been said and whether there is evidence to support the statements. You ask for her source of information, why she is making certain statements, and how she can verify what she has said so that credibility is established.

The third group of questions have to do with what is called listening with a ''third ear.'' Your purpose in asking questions in this area is to try to get the speaker to tell you those things you have a feeling haven't been said but are nevertheless important to the discussion. As you practice active listening you will become more intuitive and better able to infer from the speaker's behavior that there are hidden messages that have not yet been communicated to you.

Throughout active listening you should keep in mind that you are functioning in the role of helper; your goal is to help the speaker communicate more effectively. It is not important whether he or she uses poor grammar, speaks in half-finished sentences, stutters, stammers, laughs, or cries. What counts is that you understand what is meant in spite of environmental noise and other barriers to communication.

COMMUNICATION AND DELEGATION

If management is getting the work done through other people, then delegation is the essential to successful management. In the final analysis, the measure of a good manager is the extent to which she can assign tasks to others so that she has time to fulfill her managerial roles. Effective delegation not only allows for personal growth and development of the manager's skills, it provides opportunities for realization of the full potential of those who work under her.

If delegation is indeed such a vital part of management, why are so many nurse-managers reluctant to turn over some of their duties to their subordinates? The most obvious reason is the risk involved. The delegation of tasks and the authority to make decisions does not relieve the manager of *her* responsibility, it just lets her share that responsibility with trusted subordinates. And that leads us to another reason why nurse-managers hesitate to delegate. Many of them do not trust the workers under them. They have little or no confidence in their subordinates' competence and judgment in the performance of nursing duties. Or they may not be sure exactly how to hold their subordinates accountable for the work that they do.

There are other reasons of course. Some have to do with personal feelings of insecurity, jealous guarding of knowledge to retain expert power, and so on. But the overpowering reason has to do with a fear that a subordinate might actually do something harmful to a patient. Admittedly there is a risk in delegating tasks that have the potential for endangering the health and welfare of patients, but there is risk in any rewarding endeavor. The decision you must make is whether the risk is worth the reward. If you think it might be, then you also will want to know how to minimize the risk factor in delegation.

Assuming you are willing to sacrifice some of your peace of mind in return for more time to do the kind of work you want and need to do, let's look at some techniques you can use to delegate more effectively and with a tolerable degree of risk. A prerequisite for each of these elements of effective delegation is the ability to communicate.

know what you want done. You cannot communicate clearly and decisively if you have not encoded your message properly. You cannot tell someone else exactly what you want them to do without first being sure what the task involves. Fuzzy directives produce fuzzy responses. Give the task a name, analyze it to determine what the performer must know, do, and feel in order to carry it out as you desire; break the task down into short steps, and then communicate this to the employee.

choose your assignee carefully. Some of your employees are more experienced and better able to accept responsibility for certain tasks than others are. When you first assign a task to an employee ask for feedback. Does she know what is to be done, why, when, and how? Does she understand the task fully? Has she ever done this before? Will she need help in structuring the task so that either she or you or both can evaluate how well it is being done?

You can greatly reduce the risk of delegating if you take time to communicate with employees. It will be time well spent in terms of peace of mind because you know what is going on and whether help is needed. Once the employees are confident that they can accept responsibility for performing certain tasks and you share their confidence, you will be more willing to share the responsibility with them.

keep the feedback channels open. You and your subordinates will feel less threatened by their taking on more responsibility and making decisions if there are frequent opportunities to check up on their progress and discuss any difficulties that may have developed or to congratulate one another on how well things are going. Everyone needs to have positive feelings about what they are doing. These good feelings can be great motivators for becoming more dependable and seeking even more responsibility.

encourage development of new objectives or tasks. If when you first plunged into the risky business of delegating you chose relatively simple tasks that could be accomplished successfully, you set the stage for assigning more difficult ones. Growth usually is a gradual process, full of peaks, valleys, and plateaus, but always moving forward. It can be exciting to see employees in your unit developing new skills and to realize that as they improve and grow in their jobs you are doing the same in yours.

REFERENCES

[1]G. Goldhaber, *Organizational Communication*, (New York: Wm. C. Brown Co., 1974).

[2]R. Likert, *New patterns of Management*, (New York: McGraw-Hill Book Co., 1961).

[3]C. R. Rogers and F. J. Roethlisberger, "Barriers and gateways to communication," *Harvard Business Review*, (July-Aug., 1952).

[4]R. Harrison, "Nonverbal communication," in J. H. Cambell and H. W. Harper (eds.), *Dimensions in Communication*, (Belmont, Calif.: Wadsworth, 1970).

[5]S. A. Bower and G. H. Bower, *Asserting Yourself*, (Reading, Mass.: Addison-Wesley Pub. Co., 1976).

[6]J. Baer, *How to be an Assertive (Not Aggressive) Woman in Life, Love, and on the Job*, (Brattleboro, Vt.: The Book Press, 1976).

[7]D. Level, Jr., "Communication effectiveness: method and situation," *Journal of Business Communication*, (Fall, 1972).

[8]*Ibid.*

[9]C. Rogers and F. Roethlisberger, *op. cit.*

[10]C. R. Rogers, *On Becoming a Person*, (Boston: Houghton-Mifflin Co., 1970).

[11]R. Strebe, "Just what do you hear?" *Supervisor Nurse*, (May, 1975).

[12]W. R. Van Dersal, *The Successful Supervisor in Government and Business*, 3rd ed., (New York: Harper and Row Publishers, Inc., 1974).

SUGGESTED READINGS

J. Baer, *How to Be an Assertive (Not Aggressive) Woman in Life, Love, and on the Job*. (Brattleboro, Vt.: The Book Press, 1976).

S. A. Bower and G. H. Bower, *Asserting Yourself*, (Reading, Mass.: Addison-Wesley Pub. Co., 1976).

H. Chenevert, *Special Techniques for Assertiveness Training for Women in Health Occupations*, (St. Louis: C. V. Mosby Co., 1978).

D. L. Costley, "Basis for effective communication," *Supervisor Nurse*, (Jan., 1973).

A. J. Davis, "Body talk," *Supervisor Nurse*, (June, 1978).

A. M. De Felippo, "Big nurse: little ego," *Supervisor Nurse*, (Sept., 1978).

G. F. Donnelly, "The assertive nurse, or how to say what you mean without shaking," *Nursing '78*, (Jan., 1978).

C. Epstein, "Breaking the barriers to communications on the health team," Book selection *Nursing '74*, (Sept., 1974).

W. G. Gallagher, "Communication is everybody's business," *Supervisor Nurse*, (July, 1971).

W. V. Haney, *Communication and Organizational Behavior*, (Homewood, Ill.: Richard D. Irwin, Inc., 1973).

E. A. McConnell, "Delegation—myth or reality?" *Supervisor Nurse*, (Oct., 1979).

R. Strebe, "Just what do you hear?" *Supervisor Nurse*, (May, 1975).

E. M. Volanta, "Mastering the managerial skill of delegation," *Journal of Nursing Administration*, (Jan.-Feb., 1974).

L. Wiley. "Communications: Understanding the gravity of the situation," *Nursing '76*, (April, 1976).

chapter 8
index

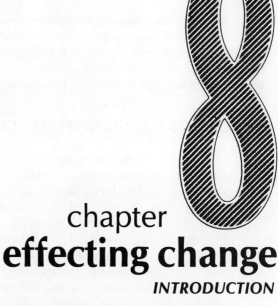

chapter
effecting change
INTRODUCTION

In many of the previous chapters of this book we have talked about change and some of the studies that have been done from the perspective of researchers in various disciplines. We have discussed such structural changes as management by objectives, decentralization and whole-task nursing for job enrichment, and behavioral change models, such as those proposed by leadership and management style theorists and situational theorists. In this chapter we will discuss planned change from the perspective of the social scientists who are change theorists.

The study of *planned change*, in contrast to *natural and unplanned change*, is relatively new. One of the first collections of studies of planned change was published in 1961 and edited by Bennis, Benne, and Chin, under the title, *The Planning of Change.*[1] Change theorists are interested in psychological and social factors that influence the success of planned change. We will discuss the role of the change agent in enhancing acceptance of change in an organizational setting. In this context, the change agent is the manager and the client system is one or more individuals in the organization.

The nature of the change and the unique characteristics are of interest to the change agent because they influence the success with which a planned change can be initiated, implemented, and maintained over a period of time. To illustrate how these and other factors contribute to the acceptance of a change for the better, we have presented an example of planned change in a health care organization.

In the final phase of the change process the acceptance of the planned change must be evaluated and validated. The manner in which this might be done is explained. Members of the client system can be motivated to continue with the planned change if creative and visible evidence of the change is presented. Some suggestions as to how this might be done are included in the last section of this chapter. Finally, there is a word about the evaluation of the performance of the change agent and a checklist that you might use to appraise your competence as a change agent.

APPROACHES TO PLANNED CHANGE

Leavitt proposed three approaches to planned change within organizations: (1) *structural* approaches which attempt to modify divisions of the work, lines of authority and centralization of power; (2) *technological* approaches which are focused on problem-solving instruments, such as the computers; and (3) *people* approaches, which attempt to directly influence the behavior of individuals within the organization.[2]

Of these three approaches, the first-line manager would probably be most effective in initiating and implementing change in people, less effective in bringing about change in structure, and least likely to be able to initiate and implement change through technology. Changes in structure are not likely to be successfully implemented and maintained, however, unless the change is accepted and sanctioned by the people who will participate in the structural change.

Most of the research in the area of planned change is being done by behavioral scientists who are concerned with the people in the change process. Bennis, a leader in change theory, developed a classification of the ways in which change can be implemented in an organization. He defined planned change as the effort to apply knowledge of the behavioral sciences to the practical problems in organizations through the use of a *deliberate and collaborative relationship between the change agent and the client system*[3] (italics mine).

In Chin's model for changing, the change agent acts in the role of helper to the client system. Goals and objectives for progress are determined cooperatively. Plans for goal achievement are developed and implemented in a cooperative and collaborative relationship.[4] To illustrate, a head nurse, as a change agent working toward more detailed nursing care plans for patients on her unit, would work with a client system composed of her staff nurses. Together they would establish objectives to accomplish the goal, implement activities, and evaluate the effectiveness of their plans for the change.

ACCEPTANCE OF CHANGE

Prior to working with the individual or group to initiate and implement a change, the change agent should attend to some psychological factors that can enhance or prevent the client system's acceptance of the change.

The people who are to implement the change must be aware of the need for it, understand what the change will entail and how it will affect them, and perceive the proposed change as being one that will bring about improvement. Additionally, and perhaps most important, they must view the change as being compatible with their own personal values and not in conflict with the policies and regulations of the organization.

Kurt Lewin, a pioneer in the study of change, developed a three-stage model for the process of change.[5] In the first stage the client system responds to environmental conditions that suggest a need for change. In experiments conducted by Lewin and his associates during World War II an attempt was made to change the buying habits of a group of housewives. The usual cuts of meat were in scarce supply during wartime, so the specific aim of the researchers was to get the women to buy the less popular organ meats such as sweetbreads, kidneys, and beef hearts.

One outcome of the study was the suggestion that people become aware of the need for change when (1) expectations are not met, (2) discomfort and guilt arise because of some action or lack of it, and (3) an obstacle to change has been removed.

When you are assessing the chances for success in implementing a change that you are considering, these motivational factors should be taken into account. Expectations are standards or criteria by which people measure performance and its outcome. The people in the client system must be aware of these expectations and consider them to be reasonable and attainable. They then, consciously or unconsciously, measure their own behavior against the criteria. If they realize that they have taken an action that does not lead to fulfillment of the expectations, or if they fail to act in such a way as to achieve what is expected of them, they will probably experience guilt and discomfort. Or, as we learned in the chapter on motivation, they may not be able to meet objectives that they consider to be desirable because of some obstacle in their path.

A head nurse who has as her objective an improvement in the recording of nursing activities and patients' responses to nursing care on source-oriented records such as nurses' notes and flow sheets, must first consider the possibility that her staff nurses do not share her concern because they are satisfied with the way they are charting. They may not realize that (1) there is a better way to document nursing activities and patient response; (2) there is a discrepancy between their performance and the ideal; (3) their current performance in record keeping can lead to poor quality patient care difficulties with accreditation of the organization, and financial problems with third party payors who do not find documented evidence that an acceptable level of nursing care is being provided.

Another concern of the head nurse in this situation should be whether her staff nurses have had sufficient orientation in the use of the printed forms on which they are expected to chart and if they have the time to chart as they should. It also is possible that some staff nurses who have been taught problem-oriented record keeping in nursing school will find source-oriented records an obstacle to charting activities and outcomes of the nursing process.

content of the change

Changes are the eventual outcome of problem-solving activities. The content of the change is the list of objectives, tasks to be performed, or plans for resolution of a problem that has been accurately defined and explicitly stated. In the process of problem solving, the change agent must gather data, analyze the information collected, identify the problems, and then prepare objectives for change.

The analysis of data is an intellectual endeavor that comes naturally to some people and is more difficult for others. Before going on with our discussion of the content of change, we will digress for a moment to clarify what is meant by analysis of data.

Bloom suggests three levels of analysis during the process of thinking:[6] (1) breaking down the whole body of information into its constituent parts and classifying the bits of information; (2) detecting and making explicit the relationships among the elements of information to determine how they are connected and how they interact; (3) recognizing how the parts are organized, their arrangement and their structure. The organizing principles thus obtained allow one to draw inferences that suggest a course of action.

Returning to our discussion of the content of change, we might consider an example of a procedural or structural change that involved people and their participation in planned change. At the beginning of this change episode it seemed that a change was needed in the performance of the staff nurses. Later, after data gathering and analysis, it was determined that the procedure had served as an obstacle to their performing as expected. Here is what happened.

The head nurse of a medical unit in an acute care facility observed that there was an increase in reported drug errors. A review of the incident reports compiled for a two-month period indicated that almost all the errors were omissions of drugs that should have been given during the hours of 7:00 and 11:00 a.m., and that the omissions were reported by three of the nurses on her staff.

A private meeting with each the three nurses resulted in a consensus that the drugs prescribed for their patients usually were not available at the time the drug errors occurred. The nurses became distracted with other duties and forgot to check later to see whether the drugs had arrived. The head nurse then met with the staff nurses as a group and together they decided that there was a need to change the method by which drugs were being ordered from the pharmacy by the ward secretary. She was asked to join the nurses and participate in deciding how the method for ordering drugs could be changed so that medications would be on hand when needed.

Objectives for the change under consideration in the above example would be focused on the procedure for ordering drugs from the pharmacy. It is not possible to change one structural variable in a complex system such as a hospital without affecting the whole system through one or more of its subsystems. In the event that the new method for ordering drugs would involve some change in the duties and responsibilities of personnel in the *hospital pharmacy*, the change agent must attend to this detail. In essence, the people in the pharmacy are incorporated into the client system and therefore are involved in the entire process. Their awareness of the need for change must be considered and their participation in preparing the change objectives encouraged.

details of the plans for change

If plans for the change are not sufficiently detailed and do not take into consideration some of the difficulties that might arise during implementation, the chances for acceptance and maintenance of the change are greatly diminished. The change agent will need to anticipate these difficulties and prepare a strategy for dealing with them. A positive outcome of this need for detailed planning is that it forces the change agent to clarify in his/her own mind the purposes, process, and expected end-results of the change. If the change agent is not able to meet resistance with clearly stated and plausible arguments in favor of the change, he/she probably will not be able to bring it about.

The accessibility of *resources* is a major detail that must be attended to in planning for change. These resources include equipment, space and facilities, and time, as well as the available people and their talents and skills. First-line managers cannot command the use of unlimited resources. By virtue of their position in the hierarchy they are limited in the resources they can procure for purposes of implementing change.

This is not to say that lack of resources will prevent making a change for the better. If people want to accomplish a goal badly enough, they will improvise, find a satisfactory substitute, or find some creative way to do what they want to do. If it is absolutely impossible to obtain or substitute for an essential resource, it is still possible to accomplish some of the objectives for change by revising the plans so that they are less ambitious and more practical. Compromises that are made in objectives and plans for achieving an important goal are not the same as a compromise of principles. People who are committed to a principle and a goal may need to make some compromises in regard to the way in which that principle can be realized and the goal achieved.

a change for the better

Members of the client system will accept change more readily if they perceive the change as one that will be personally advantageous. Everett Rogers identified this concern for personal advantage as one of five factors influencing the success of planned change. He called it *relative advantage* and suggested that whether or not the change will actually be beneficial is not as important as whether the client system *perceives* it to be so.[7]

The change agent must use care in employing tactics that deal with the client system's perception of a particular situation. Strategems frequently used to induce change by convincing people that it will be advantageous to them are called *empirical-rational* or *self-interest and persuasive* strategems. Although these may be successful in the short run, they have the potential for abuse, deceit, and betrayal of the client system's trust in the change agent. If, after the change is implemented, people find that the personal disadvantages of the change outweigh the advantages, they will no longer implement it and will return to former patterns of behavior.

People derive their perception of events in a situation from their past experiences or empirical evidence, and from rational conclusions drawn from their knowledge of the facts as they understand them. Resistance to change can occur if people do not have full information about a proposed change and therefore cannot draw rational conclusions about how it will affect them. The change agent must be able to substantiate the need for change with objective data, then share with the client system her own perception of the goals for change and their relative advantage to the client system.

One problem with the use of persuasive strategems is that it usually is difficult to plan a change that will have favorable consequences for every person involved. It is possible that some people will lose status or perhaps even their jobs; others may have an increased work load, or be assigned to unfamiliar tasks or tasks that are damaging to their self-esteem. If persuasion is used and an appeal is made to the self-interest of the group members, these approaches must be used honestly and ethically, without raising false hopes in the client system.

Members of the client system will have difficulty taking a rational stand for or against a change if they do not understand it or have not been aware that there is a better method or technique for performing a task. The change agent has responsibility for informing the client system of the details of the change and its expected benefits so that they can make a more rational decision about participating in its implementation. We frequently accuse people of being inflexible and having an inherent dislike for change when the actual cause may be either a lack of information or a dislike of the method by which a change is introduced.

compatibility of values, needs, and goals

The change agent must be familiar with the norms and customs of the client system and the rules, policies, and regulations in force in the organization in which the change is to take place. A change that people perceive to be inconsistent with their values and needs or against the rules will be resisted.

Change should not be made for personal reasons to satisfy the ego needs of the change agent. If you are ambitious and eager to impress your superiors and hope to use planned change to advance your own cause, your motivation for initiating change is at fault and you are going to meet resistance once the people in your client system figure out what is going on. A rationale for change should be based on the requirements of an individual, group or organization, *not* on the personal requirements of the change agent.

Hunt suggests that from hundreds of reports of research studies conducted by change theorists, and his own surveys of change programs, the vital relationship in the change process is between *power* and *values*.[8] Improving interpersonal relationships among members of the client system and the sensitive use of power to develop attitudes consistent with the objectives of the change are major tasks in the change process.

The concepts of power, influence and control were defined and discussed in Chapter 6. Behavioral scientists view influence and power as sources of strength for leaders which, when sensitively and humanely employed, can contribute to effective leadership and the accomplishment of goals that are important to the client system as well as to the change agent and the organization.

molding and developing values

Assuming that the philosophy and values underlying a contemplated change are not in conflict with those of the organization in which the change is to be made, the change agent will need to try to find out if the members of the client system share these same values. It is extremely difficult to measure attitude with any degree of certainty about the results. People, especially those in subordinate positions, have a tendency to say what they think the evaluator wants to hear. In a one-to-one dialogue, or a group discussion about values, you should not be surprised if your subordinates verbally express one set of values they think will be acceptable to their peers and superiors and later behave in ways that belie some of their statements. This is not so much a matter of deliberately deceiving others as it is the lack of a clear understanding of what they do believe to be valuable.

One useful technique in molding and developing values is values clarification exercises. Another is clearly communicating to the members of the client system exactly what the underlying values of a proposed change are. Are there sound reasons for making the change? How will things be better after the change than they are now? Does everyone agree that the expected outcome will be better than the status quo? What might be gained and what might be lost as a result of the change? Do gains outweigh the losses in terms of personal satisfaction and an improvement in the quality of care provided?

Communicating with others for the purpose of changing values and attitudes should be done in such a way that those who are not committed to the change will have a chance to ask questions and receive straightforward and truthful answers. We have to concede that this kind of dialogue is more time-consuming and harder to control than one-way communication, but it has the advantage of clarifying values and counteracting misperceptions.

Bobbitt et al. suggest two other techniques for attitude change through communication: (1) Give both sides of the issue. Such a technique encourages the receiver to listen more attentively to your message; (2) Argue your case using a ''nonextreme'' counter position if the person has a deep-rooted commitment to his or her position. If, however, he or she is only mildly opposed to the attitude you are advocating, then a more extreme argument for your stance is probably more productive.[9]

Behavioral scientists also believe that focusing only on attitude change without attention to actual behavior may not produce the desired results. They suggest that a change in behavior will gradually produce a change in attitude. It takes time to change behavior, but the results are more permanent in terms of attitudinal change.

An important factor in acceptance of change is whether or not members of the client system feel an *ownership of the problem* and *ownership of the decision* to make a change. A person might be aware that something ought to be done about a particular situation and yet feel no urge to participate in deciding that a change should be made and how it should be carried out. When group members accept ownership of a problem and are committed to making a change as a means of dealing with it, they are indeed entering into a collaborative relationship with one another and with the change agent. This kind of attitude is essential to the success of planned change.

The concern for values, attitudes, and ownership of the problem is not limited to the client system. As change agent, you must be fully aware of your own attitudes and interests, your skill in interpersonal relationships, and your feelings about the proposed change. If you have sufficient self-knowledge, you will be more realistic in your approach to the initiation and implementation of the change.

THE NATURE OF THE CHANGE

As we mentioned earlier, the change agent can approach organizational change by attempting to modify the behavior and attitudes of the people, and by trying to alter the structure elements of the organization. In an attempt to modify either of these variables, the change agent will need to consider the kind of change needed and the characteristics of the change.

kind of change needed

A change that is deliberately induced is done so for the purpose of improvement. Existing conditions, whatever their nature, are such that a change of some kind is indicated. During the diagnostic phase of the change process your task is to collect data and analyze it so that critical and specific needs can be identified. As a guide to the kinds of information that will be helpful, you might consider the general area or category of the need for change.

Olson presents three broad categories of the kinds of organizational change that might be indicated: (1) organizational dysfunction, (2) expansion of organizational facilities, and (3) awareness of a missing function.[10]

Dysfunction within an organization can be manifested by unsatisfactory quality or quantity output, rate of turnover of personnel, interpersonal conflict, and conflicting status relations within an organization or one of its subsystems. An example of this type of dysfunction is the problem presented when an RN assigned to the position of module leader in the modular approach to nursing care has difficulty getting cooperation from the more experienced and team-nursing oriented RN's who are supposed to work under her direction.

Expansion of facilities provided by a health-care organization is partly due to an increased demand for more sophisticated equipment and technologically advanced procedures for meeting the medical and nursing needs of patients. As an example of this kind of induced change, we might consider the plight of the head nurse of a coronary care unit in a 200-bed hospital. The number of patients admitted to the unit increased by 100 percent within a year, necessitating the addition of ten beds and more advanced monitoring equipment. A change of this kind is a major undertaking that requires the support of higher levels of management as well as alterations in each of the subsystems related to the coronary care unit.

In order to be aware of a *missing function,* the change must, of course, know what constitutes the norm for the client system and what a system or subsystem can realistically be expected to provide. The ideal patient care unit, community health agency, or home health care division is a highly desirable goal, but limitations of available money, staff, and other resources deny the realization of a utopia. There are, however, relatively simple changes that can be implemented for a gradual improvement so that the services provided are closer to the ideal. In this context, the first-line manager has many opportunities to function as change agent.

An example of a missing function that can be remedied by change in a home health care agency is the realization that elderly and physically handicapped patients might not be aware that they can request that their medications not be put in containers with child-proof caps. Incorporating this information into the component of patient education for families in which there are no small children is a minor change, but it could help minimize the frustration experienced by patients who take their own medication but have difficulty opening the containers. It also could have the added benefit of motivating the patients to comply more readily with their prescribed regimen.

characteristics of the change

In our discussion of acceptance of change we mentioned that Rogers had identified five factors that influence the success of planned change. The first two of these factors, *relative advantage* and *compatibility of values, needs, and goals* have been explained. We will now turn our attention to the remaining three factors that are related to the nature of the change and its dimensions in an organizational setting. These factors are: *complexity, divisibility,* and *communicability.*[11]

complexity

In general, the more complex the change, the less likely it is to be adopted, particularly when the change requires a high level of cognitive skills to grasp complex ideas. It is believed, however, that once a complex change has been adopted, it is more likely to persist.

Complex changes usually involve two or more variables in the organization and a large and varied client system. Examples of complex changes in an organization include the introduction of a new employee appraisal system, the implementation of management by objectives, and the change to a primary nursing care system in an organization in which the traditional team nursing or functional approach has been used.

A complex change in which the client system is an individual might be the promotion of a staff nurse to the position of head nurse. Such a change will require the learning of management theory and leadership skills on the part of the person making the change to a new position in the hierarchy.

divisibility

This characteristic refers to the ease with which a change can be tried on a small scale as a pilot project before being introduced throughout the system. This divisibility and application on a trial basis is helpful in a revision and refinement of the change and identification of environmental forces that either enhance or impede its acceptance and retention.

An example might be the introduction of a new system for the assessment of patients who are being seen for the first time in a neighborhood health clinic. Several of the nurses on the staff could try the new system for a month, evaluate its effectiveness, and recommend that it be continued as it was originally conceived, or modified slightly to improve its effectiveness, or discarded altogether.

communicability

Throughout the entire process of change that involves both the client system and the change agent, there must be frequent and open communication between and among the people engaged in the process. If a change is easily described and grasped, it will be more readily accepted and diffused throughout the client system. The change agent may use both formal and informal channels of communication to get across the details of the change and to clear up any misperceptions or misunderstandings the members of the client system might have.

AN EXAMPLE OF PLANNED CHANGE

The following is an example of one change agent's attempt to engage two of her subordinates in the process of planned change. While reading this example, try to identify some of the factors that contributed to successful implementation and maintenance of the change.

Susan Black is a charge nurse in a convalescent care unit of a large medical center. Two of her nurse attendants repeatedly "forget" to carry out some of the duties listed on their assignment sheets. When Susan asks them why the work was not done, their usual response is "you didn't remind me," or something to that effect. Susan tried without success to impress upon them the importance of accepting responsibility for carrying out assigned duties without continuous reminders to do the work.

Susan learned that this behavior was also exhibited with other charge nurses who had worked with the attendants. There were a number of forces at work pressuring Susan to make a change. Not the least of these were patient complaints about neglect and Susan's own frustration at not being able to motivate the two attendants. She decided to change the way in which the assignments were made. She planned to have the attendants complete their own assignment sheets after she had selected the patients they were to care for.

Because it was not an acute care facility and new orders for the patients were infrequently written, Susan did not view the change as being very complex. It was, however, a departure from the norm because nurse attendants at the agency were not accustomed to being allowed to participate in planning their work day. There was no policy, rule, or regulation of the agency that prohibited the change.

Having received permission from her supervisor to try the new way of completing assignment sheets for these two attendants, Susan set about creating an awareness in them of a need for change. She discussed with them their feelings about depending on her so much and helped clarify in their minds the discomfort they felt when they repeatedly turned to her for direction. She worked hard to communicate what would be involved in the change and what would be expected of them. She assured them that they would have ample time to learn their new task of completing assignment sheets and promised support and guidance during the first stages of change. They were told that she would review their "self-made" assignment sheets each day before they started the day's work. She was assertive in telling them what she wanted done and very clear and concise in her directions to them.

During the time that Susan was explaining the new system to the nurse attendants she proceeded very slowly, was careful not to seem impatient with them as they learned, and complimented them on their cooperation and willingness to give the change a try. She told them of her confidence in their ability to take on this additional task and share responsibility so she would be free to do other tasks that could not be delegated.

During the time Susan was planning the change she sought input from the nurse attendants and from her immediate supervisor. At one point she became discouraged because her supervisor questioned whether any time would be saved by having the nurse attendants fill out their own assignment sheets. Susan considered the criticism but finally decided that her goal was not to save time but to wean her attendants away from her and help them accept more responsibility and develop job maturity.

The incident with her supervisor did have a good effect, however, because it motivated Susan to think about and write down specific and sequential objectives for implementing her planned change. Some of her objectives were:

1. Conduct three 30-minute sessions with the two nurse attendants in next two weeks.

    a. First session: Attendants will be able to explain in their own words (1) *why* assignment sheets are made each day; (2) *what* should be included on an assignment sheet for a nurse attendant; and (3) *where* information for making out assignment is obtained.

    b. Second session: Given an assignment sheet with only the patient's name written in the space, nurse attendants will be able to write in all nursing and housekeeping tasks for which they will be responsible and the times each task is to be done.

    c. Third session: Attendants will be able to explain the procedure for completing assignment sheets each day and having them checked by head nurse or nurse in charge.

2. Conduct two 15-minute sessions in the third week to allow for feedback from nurse attendants and revision of objectives as indicated.

3. Begin trial period of three consecutive days during the fourth week, allowing nurse attendants to make out their own assignment sheets.

4. Follow-up session of 20 minutes during fifth week to hear nurse attendants' evaluation of their progress and provide assistance wherever needed.

Note that Susan established a time frame and deadlines for accomplishment of certain objectives. She presented the objectives to the nurse attendants and asked for suggestions for change and revision.

Eight weeks after identifying her problem, planning the change, and implementing it, Susan was happy to see that it was accepted and working. The time spent in having the nurse attendants fill out their own assignment sheets was more than compensated for by the time saved when they no longer waited for reminders from her.

VALIDATION OF ACCEPTANCE OF PLANNED CHANGE

Your ultimate goal in your role as change agent is independent of the client system and maintenance of the change. If you do a good job of effecting the change, you will not be needed by your client system to carry on with the improved method, behavior, or whatever. A change that is accepted and internalized by the client system should be integrated into its own value system.

Acceptance of change does not always mean that the final change has not undergone some revision and that plans and objectives have not been adapted to the situation. Flexibility is essential to the success of planned change. The ideal rarely is achieved, but progress toward the ideal can be accomplished. That is not to say that the integrity of the change should be compromised. The more realistic the expectations for planned change, the closer the final outcome will be to the ideal.

Determination of progress toward the acceptance of change is twofold. It should include an *ongoing evaluation* or assessment of things as they are at any given point during the process, and *a final or terminal appraisal* of the situation as it exists at the final phase of validation. It is apparent that some time limits must be set for the performance of activities in each phase and that a termination point is established for the process. The established time frames help set limits and provide motivation for doing whatever must be done to bring about the planned change.

The techniques and tools that you will use for an ongoing evaluation and for terminal validation are essentially the same. They differ in the time they are used, that is, at what phase of the process, and whether the benchmarks used for the appraisal are future-oriented objectives or present-oriented outcomes. In the following pages we will examine two categories of evaluation tools and instruments by which the process can be evaluated: (1) analysis of driving and restraining forces, and (2) data collection and presentation of evidence of change.

analysis of driving and restraining forces

In Lewin's three-stage model for change, two kinds of forces affecting change are considered. These forces are operant in both the unfreezing and refreezing stages. The forces in favor of and facilitating movement toward change are called the *driving forces*. Those forces which impede progress toward the desired change are called *restraining forces*.

As an example of the analysis of driving and restraining forces, consider this situation in which a new system for the administration of medications was introduced on a patient care unit. The old system used unit-dose drugs sent from the pharmacy department and administered by members of a medication team. This applied only to medications given regularly: "stat" doses and "prn" medications were given by staff nurses assigned to specific patients.

The proposed system required elimination of the medication team, shifting responsibility for administration of all medications to the staff nurses who were RN's and LPN's. Drugs would still be sent up in unit doses from the pharmacy and placed on medication carts as they were under the old system.

Driving forces for change were:

1. There was no change in the pharmacy's mode of operation.
2. Higher levels of management were informed of the proposed change and gave their approval.
3. Patients would benefit from a less fragmented delivery of nursing care.
4. Staff nurses would be better informed about medications their patients were receiving and more alert to adverse reactions, side effects, etc.
5. The likelihood of drug errors, harmful drug interactions and drug-food interactions should be diminished.

6. Nurses formerly assigned to medication teams would be available for modular nursing and the sharing of responsibility for total patient care.

Restraining forces were:

1. There was no opportunity for input in the decision to make the change by the staff nurses.
2. Staff nurses were informed of the nature of the change, but did not take part in planning for it.
3. There were too few medication carts, the result being that at times there would be three or more persons attempting to use them, causing delays and frustration in the administration of medications.
4. The medication carts that were available were not designed so that more than one person could use a cart efficiently.
5. There were only two occasions on which the staff nurses were consulted to determine how the change was working.
6. The change was implemented on all three shifts rather than on one shift on a trial basis and at a time when help might be available for solving any problems that might arise.
7. No notice was taken of the implied threat of loss of job and perhaps status for the nurses on the medication team.

The data obtained from an analysis of these forces would be helpful at the time strategies for change are being selected rather than after the implementation phase. It would still be possible, however, to look back into the process and make another start, beginning at the phase of awareness of need for change. In any case, one purpose of such an analysis would be to determine the best ways to strengthen the driving forces and weaken the restraining forces. Another would be to determine the best time to use the strengthening and weakening strategies so that they will be more effective. There often are optimal times when forces in favor of change can be used most effectively.

Bennis, et al. caution the change agent against increasing the driving forces only. Such one-sided effort will result in a reactive increase in the restraining forces.[12] In the example presented above, driving forces could have been strengthened by:

• Holding group meetings to discuss the benefits of the proposed change.
• Providing opportunities for values clarification and molding of attitudes consistent with values of the change.

- Asking staff nurses to identify disadvantages of the old system.

  Restraining forces could have been weakened by:

- Providing opportunities for participative decision-making by the staff nurses.
- Allowing for input from staff nurses during all phases of the process.
- Setting up a trial run for one group in the client system before diffusing the change.
- Providing adequate equipment for implementation of the change.
- Holding meetings for ventilation of feelings and expression of thoughts about the change. In short, providing a safety valve for the restraining forces.
- Utilizing the problem-solving process for dealing with restraining forces.

data collection and presentation of evidence

There are multiple ways to collect data and present documented evidence of change. Examples of these techniques and tools abound in every aspect of our lives. With a sound understanding of the meanings of relevance, reliability, and validity in the presentation of data, the creative change agent is limited only by her own creativity and that of the members of the client system. The selection and utilization of procedures and techniques for data collection and presentation of evidence might include:

- Survey of members of the client system and any others affected by the change.
- First-hand observation of changed behavior and other signs of change.
- Group discussions to obtain feedback.
- One-to-one dialogues to obtain feedback.
- Compilation of verbal and written comments from patients, colleagues, and others who have personally experienced benefit from the change or have seen evidence of the benefits in the lives of others.
- Visual representation of progress, including photographs of "before and after" charts, graphs, and other depictions of progress and gain.

There are motivational advantages in the use of these and similar techniques in addition to their applicability to the task of validating acceptance of change. People like being a part of a successful team effort. They want to feel good about themselves and the people with whom they have worked to bring about a change for the better.

EVALUATION OF THE CHANGE AGENT'S PERFORMANCE

In her description of a successful change agent; Janet Rodgers identifies *interpersonal competence* as the most significant skill.[13] Such competence demands a capacity to involve others in setting goals and planning for their achievement in a changing environment. The competent change agent is sensitive to the needs and values of the client system, aware of the many variables in any situation, and flexible enough to deal with the variables on a contingency basis.

Self-knowledge is a valuable asset to the change agent in terms of her ability and willingness to initiate change and promote growth in herself as well as in the client system. A checklist such as the one shown in Figure 8-1

figure 8.1   checklist for evaluating change agent's performance

1. Identified and validated the need for change.

2. Created in the client system an awareness of the need for change.

3. Established ownership of the problem.

4. Diagnosed general kind of change needed, in collaboration with client system.

5. Considered factors affecting success of planned change.

6. Prepared explicit objectives for change with input from members of the client system.

7. Selected strategies for change on basis of existing situational factors.

8. Applied strategies using continual feedback for assessment of their effectiveness.

9. Revised plans as indicated by data obtained through feedback.

10. Used creativity in designing instruments to collect data for purposes of validation and preservation of evidence of acceptance of change.

11. Used problem-solving techniques throughout process.

12. Employed interpersonal skills to motivate and support client system throughout process.

may be used as a starting point to enhance your awareness of personal strengths and weaknesses and serve as a guide for continued growth.

REFERENCES

[1]W. G. Bennis, K. D. Benne and R. Chin (eds.), *The Planning of Change*, (New York: Holt, Rinehart and Winston, 1969).

[2]H. J. Leavitt, "Applied organizational change in industry: Structured, technological and humanistic approaches," in S. March (ed.), *Handbook of Organizations*, (Chicago: Rand McNally, 1965).

[3]W. G. Bennis, *Changing Organizations*, (New York: McGraw-Hill Book Co., 1966).

[4]R. Chin, "The utility of systems models and developmental models for practitioners," In E. Maccoby (ed.), *The Planning of Change: Readings in the Behavioral Sciences*, (New York: Holt, Rinehart and Winston, 1958).

[5]K. Lewin, "Group decisions and social change," In E. Maccoby (ed.), *Readings in Social Psychology*, 3rd ed. (New York: Holt, Rinehart, and Winston, 1968).

[6]B. S. Bloom, *The Taxonomy of Educational Objectives*, (New York: Longmans, Green, 1954), p. 144.

[7]E. Rogers, *Diffusion of Innovation*, (New York: The Free Press of Glenco, 1962).

[8]J. W. Hunt, *The Restless Organization*, (Sidney, Australia: John Wiley & Sons, Australia Pty. Ltd, 1972).

[9]H. R. Bobbitt, Jr., et al., *Organizational Behavior*, (Englewood Cliffs: Prentice-Hall, Inc., 1974).

[10]E. M. Olson, "Strategies and techniques for the nurse change agent," *Nursing Clinics of North America*, (June, 1979).

[11]E. Rogers, *op. cit.*

[12]W. G. Bennis, K. D. Benne, and R. Chin, *op. cit.*

[13]J. Rodgers, "Theoretical considerations involved in the process of change," *Nursing Forum*, (Vol. 12, no. 2 1973), p. 161.

SUGGESTED READINGS

E. S. Asprec, "The process of change," *Supervisor Nurse*, (Oct., 1975).

A. J. Brown, "Change in charting on critical care units," *Nursing Clinics of North America*, (June, 1979).

J. Deal, "The timing of change," *Supervisor Nurse*, (Feb. 1977).

L. P. Dean, "The change from functional to primary nursing," *Nursing Clinics of North America*, (June, 1979).

H. Gasset, "Participative planned change," *Supervisor Nurse*, (March, 1976).

A. L. Hofing, et al., "The importance of maintenance in implementing change," *Journal of Nursing Administration*, (Dec., 1979).

J. Kriegel, "People are not resistant to change," *Supervisor Nurse*, (Nov., 1971).

A. Levenstein, "Effective change requires change agent," *Journal of Nursing Administration*, (June, 1979).

A. Marriner, "Behavioral aspects of planned change," *Supervisor Nurse*, (Dec., 1977).

M. Miller, "Task force: genesis of change," *Nursing Clinics of North America*, (June, 1979).

H. Mizer and A. Barraro, "Change: for nursing service and education," *Nursing Clinics of North America*, June, 1979).

J. Rodgers, "Theoretical considerations involved in the process of change," *Nursing Forum*, (Vol. 12 no. 2, 1973).

B. J. Stevens, "Effecting change," *Journal of Nursing Administration*, (Feb., 1975).

L. B. Welch, "Planned change in nursing: The theory," *Nursing Clinics of North America*, (June, 1979).

L. Wiley, "Tips for the timid or how can one little nurse hope to change the rules?" *Nursing '76*, (May, 1976).

chapter 9
index

chapter 9

dealing with conflict and handling grievances

INTRODUCTION

General systems theory suggests that an open system is continually making adaptive change in response to elements in its internal and external environment. You are familiar with the concept of homeostatis and adaptive physiologic change to maintain a steady state of equilibrium. In this chapter we will be concerned with psychosocial adaptation to conflict in the environment in which people work. As you know, failure of the human body to respond appropriately to stimuli in its internal and external environment is destructive to its physical health. In an organizational setting, inappropriate response to the conflict that is inevitable in a complex and highly diversified system can be similarly unhealthy for the organization and for the individuals and groups within the system. A major concern of managers is reduction of conflict and tension to a tolerable level and the channeling of the energy created by conflict into more constructive behavior.

Conflict theorists suggest that the cycle of conflict-adaptive change-conflict can best be dealt with if conflict is viewed as separate episodes, each of which has its own unique characteristics. By analyzing a situation and identifying the source and type of conflict, the manager is able to select approaches that are most likely to lead to reduction of the conflict and the setting of goals for problem resolution.

We will discuss some of these approaches to the resolution of particular conflict episodes and identify some tools and techniques you might use. These include confrontation, mutual problem-solving activities, and the setting of superordinate goals.

175

The last section of this chapter is devoted to a discussion of grievances and formal complaints and the procedures for handling them. Grievance procedures are helpful to both management and labor because they clearly state how employees should register legitimate complaints about organization practice and policy, and they define the manner in which management should respond to those complaints.

THE NATURE OF CONFLICT — DEFINITIONS, SOURCES, AND TYPES

Webster defines conflict as "a clash, competition, or mutual interference of opposing incompatibilities, forces, or qualities (as ideas, interests, wills)."[1] In the literature there are many variations and amplifications of this basic definition, but it is generally agreed that at the bottom of any kind of human conflict are differences or incompatibilities in the value systems of the parties involved. From these basic values people derive their opinions about what should be done, who should do it, and how it could be done most effectively.

Confusion about the role of a teacher, professional nurse, nurse-manager, or other person functioning in a structured system creates conflict because of varying expectations about the duties and responsibilities the person should assume.[2] There is ample evidence in our health care system that conflict arises because people do not perceive the same situation in exactly the same way. Individual differences in values, abilities, interests, ambitions, needs, and cultural, religious, and educational background bring about differences in the way a situation is perceived.

In his analysis of conflict, Smith[3] agrees with the notion that conflict is the result of basic differences in interests and goals and the diversity of perceptions. He studied intraorganizational conflict and from his analysis derived yet another potential source of conflict: communication.

phases of a conflict episode

In every situation in which human beings interact with one another there will be the makings of a conflict. Before we look at the kinds of disagreements and incompatibilities that can develop when people work together to accomplish a set of goals, we will consider the stages of conflict in a particular conflict episode.

In his analysis of organizational conflict Louis Pondy[4] identified five sequential steps that evolve in any given situation. His model represents the *typical* phases of conflict; not every person in the situation will experience every phase. The process begins with the aftermath of a preceding conflict episode. In a dynamic society there is a kind of chain reaction taking place. The resolution of one conflict episode only sets the stage for another.

In the first phase there are antecedent or underlying conditions in the immediate environment. This phase is called *latent conflict*. The antecedent conditions include such factors as scarcity of resources, drives for autonomy, and divergence of subgoals.

In the second phase some of the people become aware of the presence of these factors in their environment and they perceive them to be in conflict with their own goals, needs, and interests. Members of a nursing staff who wish to function with more autonomy in making decisions about nursing care perceive conflict when their nursing supervisor insists that there must be a written order by the physician for every treatment and nursing procedure performed by the nurses. Because of their awareness of the elements of conflict in this situation, the professional nurses who desire more autonomy are in the phase of *perceived conflict*.

As might be expected, people who perceive differences between their own opinions and those of others react emotionally to the situation and become angry, anxious, tense, or hostile. This phase is called *felt conflict*.

In the fourth phase, the feelings are manifested by overt behavior. During this phase of manifest conflict behavior can range from apathy to passive resistance to open aggression. Consciously or unconsciously they set out to frustrate the opposition and prevent them from reaching their goals.

The process of conflict is natural and ongoing. Management of a particular conflict episode requires intervention at strategic points to bring the situation under control and to direct the energy generated by conflict into more productive channels.

The intervention is planned according to the kind of conflict that is developing and how it is felt and manifested by the people involved.

typology and sources

Lewis proposes three main categories of human conflict: (1) *intrapersonal conflict* occurring within an individual; (2) *interpersonal conflict* between two or more persons; and (3) *intergroup conflict*.[5] To these we will add a fourth: *individual-organizational conflict* or *professional-bureaucratic conflict*.

intrapersonal conflict

We are all familiar with this kind of discord and tension within ourselves when we encounter conflict in our dealings with family, friends, subordinates, peers, and supervisors. According to Wohlking,[6] as cited in Lewis' article, intrapersonal conflict occurs when a person (1) is motivated to choose more than one alternative action, (2) is unable to make a decision because of insufficient information, or (3) feels allegiance to each of two conflicting groups.

You probably have experienced *motivational conflict* when you felt a need to delegate some managerial tasks to one of your subordinates. You are motivated to delegate because you want the subordinate to grow in her job and develop her potential and you certainly could use the free time to attend to tasks that cannot be delegated. But you also are unsure about the consequences of delegation and a little fearful of the risks involved.

Rational decision making requires the availability of sufficient data before choosing among alternatives. *Choice conflict*, as this is called, occurs because a person does not have the information she thinks she needs to choose wisely. If you do not know the level of competence at which each of your subordinates can work, you might experience some choice conflict each time you make assignments.

Conflicting allegiances can arise from expectations people have about the role of the head nurse or charge nurse. A first-line manager is in a conflict situation in regard to role expectations because she is in the middle, between her superiors and her subordinates. Your superiors expect you to represent management to your subordinates. You are the manager who is in continual contact with them. You act as interpreter of the policies and goals of the organization and are expected to enforce its rules and regulations.

At the same time, your subordinates have the right to expect you to be their representative in confrontations with higher levels of management. As their immediate supervisor you can see first hand the kinds of problems they face; they believe you should be able to see their side of the issue.

The *conflict of allegiance* is one of divided loyalty; to the organization and to the individuals who are a part of the organization. Conflict of this kind can rarely be resolved by compromise. In each situation of conflicting allegiance you must constantly be on guard against damaging your own personal integrity and that of your staff and the organization as a whole. Only you can decide the position you wish to take in a given situation. Once you have taken that position you should relinquish it only if there are compelling reasons why you should do so. Vacillating between two sides of an issue can be very demoralizing for yourself and your subordinates.

interpersonal conflict

There actually are two subcategories in this kind of conflict. One, conflict between two persons, usually arises from what is popularly called a "personality clash." For any number of reasons two people who must depend on each other to carry out certain functions cannot work together effectively. They may perceive each of their roles differently or have incompatible values and personal needs.

In the second kind of interpersonal conflict, a *group* may be divided by differences among the various members. They often can agree on goals but disagree on how to reach their goals. Members of a group who have worked together over a period of time, communicated effectively, and had some success in achieving mutual goals are better able to deal with *intragroup* conflict than those of a newly formed group who have not yet matured to this level of collaboration and cooperation.

intergroup conflict

An organization is not simply a collection of individuals doing their own thing. It is a system made up of subsystems organized for purposes of dividing the work and coordinating tasks. These subsystems must depend on one another, and their activities coordinated, if the organization is to survive. Intergroup conflict that is not resolved can do great damage to the organization.

The three major sources of intergroup conflict have been classified by Raven and Kruglanski as (1) incompatibility in goals, (2) incompatibility in subgoals, and (3) incompatibility in the means by which a shared goal can be reached.[7]

Incompatibility in goals develops when two persons or groups want the same object that *cannot be shared*. The commodity in limited supply might be material resources, status, power, personnel, or any combination of these. It is fairly easy to think of examples in which limited space creates conflict because two people want to occupy it at the same time. A head nurse wants to use a room adjacent to the nurses' station as her office. Her supervisor, or the physician, or someone from another department wants the same space for his or her own purposes.

Conflict arising from both people wanting to occupy the same *position of status* within an organization may not be so easily identified. Some people have "hidden agendas" for attaining status and power and they may use subversive means to accomplish their goals.

For example, a nurse may want the job of head nurse because she thinks she is better qualified than the person occupying that position. She may or may not be correct in her perception of the situation, but at any rate she chooses not to bring the conflict out into the open. Instead, she passively resists the head nurse in accomplishing *her* goals and offers no help in solving problems or making decisions that would contribute to a smoother running patient care unit.

Incompatibility in subgoals has to do with the delegation of tasks for the purpose of coordinating or organizing the activities of groups sharing a common goal. Essentially, the disagreement is over the division of work among various departments with the organization; as, for example, the dietary department, pharmacy, and nursing department.

Conflict in subgoals may, however, arise within a department or subsystem, as, for example, when there is disagreement among the personnel working on each of the three shifts. Nurses are all too familiar with this kind of conflict, having frequently heard the evening nurses ask, "Why can't the night shift do that?" or the day shift ask the same of the evening shift, and so on.

The third subtype of intergroup conflict, called *means/goal conflict*, occurs when groups or individuals lack the appropriate means to attain desired goals. Obstacles in their paths create frustration and a sense of helplessness. Nurse-managers who want to provide nursing care that meets the standards set by the American Nurses Association may have difficulty because of a lack of resources at their disposal.

To illustrate, as head nurse you may do all in your power to improve the competence of your subordinates and still not be successful because you do not have enough professional personnel to help with teaching, or adequate equipment, space and time to upgrade staff competence. In order to resolve the conflict you may choose confrontation, compromise, and several other techniques. Your objective may be to substitute quality for quantity by asking for two more highly trained staff members to replace four who are incompetent and unproductive.

individual-organization conflict

This fourth general type of conflict occurs when there is discord between a professional person and the organization in which she is employed. Kramer and Schmalenberg[8] call this type of discord *professional-bureaucratic* conflict, and point out that it arises from an incompatibility of role expectations. The professional nurse encounters conflict when the bureaucratic structure of the nurse-employing agency expects to exert control over her nursing activities, while at the same time nursing ideology and the nursing care standards of her professional organizations expect her to exercise some degree of autonomy in the practice of her profession.

The complexity of this type of conflict and its implications for nurse-administrators and managers cannot be ignored. It is not within the scope of this text to discuss in great depth a conflict that is so highly complex and so pervasive. It is imperative, however, that the head nurse, who is herself a part of the bureaucratic system and at the same time a professional nurse, be fully aware of the nature of the conflict and its potential for either improving patient care or diminishing its quality.

Resolution of individual-organization or professional-bureaucratic conflict in the practice of nursing will require adjustments in the health care organizations themselves. Organizations patterned after a traditional hierarchical structure follow the belief that an organization achieves its goals most effectively through the strict performance of preordained procedures and adherence to the rules and regulations it imposes on its subsystems.[9] The traditional structure will have to give way to more humanistic modes of management which will allow professionals the latitude they need to fulfill their expanded roles. Studies have shown that clarifying roles and granting nurses the freedom to practice their profession with a greater degree of independence and autonomy have a significant positive relationship with job satisfaction, lower turnover rates, and a higher level of patient care.[10]

Additionally, a satisfactory resolution of professional-bureaucratic conflict will require some degree of compromise, agreements, and conciliation on the part of nurses. The diversity of professional and personal interests, goals, and subgoals demands continued communication and negotiation. This is true of any type of conflict that a nurse-manager finds herself engaged in. The following words of Madeleine Leininger serve as excellent guidelines for a manager of conflict, regardless of the situation.

> We cannot always have and get what we want in the exact way we want it. There has to be some give and take in any conflict resolution state. However, we must not compromise easily or readily. . . . To yield professional values, ethics, major goals, or aspirations may have serious consequences.[11]

CONSTRUCTIVE AND DESTRUCTIVE CONFLICT

Newer theories of management are based on the belief that conflict is inevitable in any viable and progressive organization. Kast and Rosenzweig state that conflict is not only inevitable, but "an important, positive phenomenon in society."[12] Likert views conflict and differences of opinion as stimulants to new and better objectives and methods.[13] He prefers to view the problem of conflict as being one of how to deal with it constructively rather than one of how to suppress or eliminate it.

Interactionists such as Robbins go one step further and propose that conflict is absolutely necessary for change and growth.[14] They view stable and harmonious situations as stagnant, lacking the conditions necessary for creativity and growth. They suggest, therefore, that conflict management requires stimulation of conflict where none is evident as well as resolution of conflict that has the potential for becoming destructive.

functional or constructive conflict

Conflict is neither good nor bad; it is simply a fact of life. Whether conflict becomes functional (constructive) or dysfunctional (destructive) depends on how intense it is and how it is affecting the people involved. Lewis[15] recommends that we visualize conflict on a continuum ranging from too much or too little. The challenge to managers is to determine the point at which conflict is functional.

A tolerable level of conflict can have the following positive or constructive functions:

It can clear the air, providing a kind of safety valve for the release of pent-up emotions. Just being able to bring differences of opinion out into the open can help reduce emotionalism and lead to more rational discussion of the issue causing the conflict.

It can lead to the discovery of better alternatives for decision making, and can facilitate identification of issues and problems, when handled skillfully and constructively.

Intergroup conflict tends to bind each group's members closely together; or, it can bind rival groups when they are threatened by a common enemy. A reasonable amount of conflict and competition between two nursing care teams can be used constructively to develop team spirit and improve the effectiveness of each. At the same time, both teams can profess allegiance to one another because of their mutual opposition to the ravages of disease.

Conflict can stimulate the generation of new ideas for more innovative approaches to long-standing problems. Although change itself creates conflict, there would be no change for the better if there were not some discomfort and an awareness of the disparity between desired goals and the status quo.

dysfunctional or destructive conflict

Since conflict is expected in every viable situation, and even desirable in some, you will need to use some criteria for judging whether a conflict episode is constructive or destructive. The critical question is, of course, whether nursing productivity is being adversely affected. More specifically, you might ask yourself the following evaluative questions as suggested by deLodzia and Greenlaugh.[16]

Are people who are not originally involved in the conflict being dragged into the fray against their better judgment? If so, you must support them in their desire to remain neutral. They have a right to stay clear of the conflict and you will be able better to deal with it if fewer people are involved. As a conflict expands, it escalates and becomes more complex and difficult to manage.

Is interpersonal or intergroup conflict disrupting teamwork so that staff members are working against one another? One of the elements of conflict is the *interdependence* of the parties concerned. No member of an organization works in a vacuum and certainly not the members of a nursing staff. When there is evidence that conflict is preventing a unified group effort, it is being destructive.

Are energy and time that should be spent on patient care being diverted to political maneuvering to win support and frustrate the goals of the opposition? Taking time away from patient care to indulge in petty warfare cannot be tolerated. The sooner the conflict is resolved the sooner everyone can get on with the business of nursing.

APPROACHES TO CONFLICT RESOLUTION

There are several ways to approach a problem of conflict and resolve it in a creative and productive manner. Some are more traditional than others and therefore may be more familiar to you because you have had experience with them. The newer approaches are based on assumptions that we have already discussed. These assumptions are as follows: (1) conflict is a natural phenomenon and therefore is to be expected; (2) it may be functional or dysfunctional; (3) it can be dealt with more easily when placed in the context of a single episode with discernible phases; and (4) the conditions under which a particular conflict episode develops and is manifested will dictate the approach, techniques, and strategies selected for resolution.

In the 1930's Mary Parker Follett proposed three major paths to resolution of conflict: *domination, compromise, and integration.*[17] Since that time these approaches have been expanded and incorporated into a more comprehensive and systematic approach that is based on the concepts of participative and contingency management. This systematic or contingency approach requires analytic skills for assessment of the episode and identification of the issue or problem that is at the heart of the conflict; and the application of interpersonal and communication skills to successfully intervene and bring the conflict to a satisfactory resolution.

Domination and compromise are viable approaches under certain conditions. We will begin with a discussion of these two general paths to conflict resolution, then briefly discuss the concept of integration.

domination

Another name for this method of handling conflict is *bureaucratic resolution*. Force of authoritative power is employed to impose a solution that has been decided upon by superiors in the organization. You might choose this method in a critical conflict episode in which interpersonal differences between two people or between one individual and a group are interfering with the delivery of patient care services.

The use of coercive power is distasteful to people who believe in democratic and egalitarian problem solving and decision making. It is, nevertheless, sometimes necessary and the most effective approach when there are irreconcilable differences in personalities or in personal needs. It is least effective in resolving intergroup and intragroup conflict. The suppression of group conflict by the imposition of rules and regulations may work for a short while, but the discord will eventually return in another episode.

If you have valid and documented evidence that a staff member is creating dissension in a group or is manifesting conflict behavior that is harmful to patients, you should try to resolve the conflict through persuasion and the use of interpersonal and problem-solving skills. If these techniques fail, you may have no alternative other than using your authoritative position to resolve the problem. This may mean recommending that the employee be transferred to another area or that her employment be terminated.

compromise

The resolution of conflict by compromise or bargaining requires that each side give up something in return for something else that is wanted or needed. The outcome is not totally satisfying for either party, but it does meet at least some of their needs and reduce tension.

The agreement reached through bargaining may or may not be legally binding. In a *verbal* agreement the pressures of ethics and morality are brought to bear to ensure that each side will keep its word. *Written* contracts between labor and management are negotiated through collective bargaining; they are legally binding. Collective bargaining is discussed later in this chapter. For the present we will discuss verbal compromise negotiated by the head nurse.

Veninga[18] suggests that the manager who chooses this approach to conflict resolution must have a sense of timing and some awareness of the attitudes and goals of the opposing individuals or groups. For maximum satisfaction of their needs she should intervene only when both sides appear to be in a compromising mood, that is, when they both seem willing to find a solution rather than find fault with and blaming each other.

The least desirable time to intervene and attempt bargaining is when both sides are convinced they are in the right and have as their goal total victory over the opposition. If compromise is attempted in this kind of emotional climate it probably will fail and could even intensify the conflict by polarizing the opposing sides. Blake and Mouton, who have spent considerable time analyzing intergroup conflict in organizations, describe this polarization as a *win-lose conflict*. They write:

> The win-lose trap is for all practical purposes a foolproof structure. The capacity for empathy between victor and vanquished seems lost. They simply cannot understand each other.[19]

The techniques to use while negotiating a compromise or conciliation will be reviewed later under the topic of confrontation.

Collective bargaining or *contracting* is a term used in labor-management relations to connote a collected or united action by employees for purposes of handling grievances and negotiating contracts. Collective bargaining in nursing is still not accepted by all professional nurses as a means for improving their status in an employment setting. However, the *predisposition* of many nurses toward collective action as a legitimate and ethical approach to organizational problem solving has been shown to be related to frustrated desires for autonomy and self-control.[20] In short, professional nurses encountering professional-bureaucratic conflict in acute care facilities are inclined to resort to collective action if necessary to accomplish their goals of autonomy in the practice of their profession.

Additionally, many professional nurses and their leaders believe that improvement in economic status will ultimately have a positive effect on the quality of patient care through greater job satisfaction among nurses. This premise, though widely held, still lacks sufficient empirical testing and validation. There is little doubt, however, that having opportunities to be self-directed is related to job satisfaction and ultimately to better nursing care.

implications for the first-line manager

As an individual person and member of the nursing profession you may agree or disagree with those who believe that the quality of patient care and the economic status of nurses providing that care are directly related. Your beliefs will, of course, affect your decisions about being actively engaged in bargaining activities of the professional organizations to which you belong. As a head nurse, however, you cannot ignore the implications of the relationship between environmental working conditions and professional nurses' inclination toward collective bargaining.

The work environment of your subordinates is controlled in part by you, their head nurse. Staffing patterns and the division of work are primarily your responsibility. The professional nurses on your staff who prefer the whole-task system of work organization will experience fewer episodes of professional-bureaucratic conflict if either modular or primary nursing or a combination of the two is used instead of team nursing and other patterns that contribute to fragmentation of nursing care. When the nurses on your staff do exercise autonomy in decision making for the sake of better patient care you should be prepared to stand behind their decisions.

In all of your dealings with either professional or paraprofessional employees you must be firm and fair. But successful conflict management goes beyond this simple dictum to knowledgeable intervention. Being kind and gentle to a sick person isn't enough and being firm and fair with an employee who has a grievance won't resolve the conflict. If you are able to manage specific conflict episodes in a constructive and enlightened manner, you may prevent their escalation into formal grievance procedures, negotiations with union representatives, threats of a passive "sit-in," an organized strike, or other kinds of formal protest.

integration

This approach to conflict resolution plays down domination and compromise and focuses on a joint problem-solving effort on the part of conflicting groups or subsystems in the organization. Its ultimate purpose is the integration of each group's values into the values of the total system, and that is one of the greatest challenges administrators and managers must face.

In addition to the sharing of common values, the integrative approach also looks to the activities within an organization, particularly those concerned with problem solving and communication. It considers the variables of organizational values and structure, group behavior and attitudes, and individual needs, interests, attitudes and behavior. It is a global, all-encompassing approach to the concept of organizational conflict and its resolution. This approach must be understood by managers at all levels in the organization. It is the broad base from which theories are formulated and the systematic contingency approach to conflict has been developed.

systematic approach

The management of specific conflict episodes is not beyond the realm of first-line managers. In fact, it is very likely that many internal organizational conflicts can be more effectively managed at this level than at any other.

You are familiar with the systematic approach because you use it to resolve nursing care problems. Consider for a moment an analogy between management of the nursing care of a patient with an electrolyte imbalance and the management of conflict involving one employee or a group of subordinates.

Both the nurse at the bedside and the nurse-manager dealing with her subordinates have access to a continual flow of information about the status of their "clients." In one instance the focus of attention is the patient, in the other it is an individual or group of subordinates. The nurse provides nursing care on a contingency basis, using a variety of techniques and skills to intervene and help restore physiologic balance in the patient's internal environment, that is, the body fluids. Additionally, she uses interpersonal skills to maintain the patient's psychosocial equilibrium.

The nurse-manager also manages conflict on a contingency basis. Her concern is not primarily the physiologic needs of the participants in the conflict, though this may be relevant in some conflict episodes, but rather the psychosocial needs of employees and the productivity needs of the organization and its clients.

A systematic approach to conflict resolution is based on the concept of conflict as process. Within a particular conflict episode there are phases or stages. These stages are experienced by people who feel uncomfortable because of incompatibilities of one kind or another. The task of the manager is to determine the best time for intervention and the most effective techniques to use at any particular point of entry into the process.

The nurse who provides systematic nursing care to restore balance and homeostasis in her patient uses a broad base of knowledge and a wide variety of nursing techniques. She selects and employs the techniques that are appropriate to the situation and the patient's needs. The nurse-manager has as her goal the restoration of a harmonious balance in a conflict situation. She also employs knowledge, techniques and skills appropriate to the particular situation. She considers the nature of the conflict, the needs of the conflict participants, and the goals of the organization. Throughout the process she is aware that all the objectives for conflict resolution probably cannot be met.

Some of the techniques and tools for resolution of conflict, such as those used in dominance and compromise, have already been mentioned. Others to be discussed in the following pages include confrontation, collaborative problem solving and decision making, setting superordinate goals, and changing behavior patterns.

TECHNIQUES FOR RESOLVING CONFLICT

confrontation

A confrontation brings people together to face an issue, identify the problem, and work toward its resolution. The purpose is to clarify the problem, *not* to look for someone or something to blame for the conflict. It is the problem that must be attacked, *not* one another, higher levels of management, or the organization.

When you are involved in a confrontation you should keep four objectives clearly in mind. They are (1) to clarify the problem or issue, (2) to help establish ownership of the problem, (3) to generate open and honest communication and dialogue, and (4) to set the stage for collaborative problem solving and decision making.

guidelines for the first-line manager

A confrontation has emotional overtones that can get in the way of progress toward resolution of the conflict. Whenever you are involved in a confrontation with subordinates, peers, or higher level managers you must work at behaving assertively, positively, and rationally. Creative conflict management demands that you *act* judiciously and fairly and avoid *reacting* defensively and emotionally.

Resolve your own intrapersonal conflicts about the confrontation and its objectives. Myrtle and Glogow[21] point out that intrapersonal conflict has interpersonal effects. When resolution of your intrapersonal conflict results in increased understanding, self-assurance, and personal growth, you are more likely to be effective in dealing with others, both as individuals and in teams. If you feel good about yourself and the decisions you have made, you will be better able to help others deal more effectively with interpersonal and team relationships.

Plan the confrontation in as detailed a manner as you can before it takes place. Think about the problem and organize the information you have. If you lack sufficient information, determine what you and the other participants need to know in order to identify the problem. You can behave more assertively and rationally if you are prepared for the confrontation.

Keep the issue clearly defined and in focus. Discussion must be relevant to the information; evaluate the information being shared on the basis of whether it really contributes to identification of the specific problem. Statements that lead the discussion away from or cloud the original issue are irrelevant and distracting. They may be important to another peripheral conflict episode, but you should try to deal with only one issue at a time.

The creative management of conflict allows for ventilation of feelings, but emotionalism is not appropriate during a rational discussion. If one or more persons becomes defensive, angry, or distraught during confrontation, it probably would be best to postpone further attempts to define the issue until after participants have had time to ventilate. During the cooling off period they should try to clarify the issue in their own minds. Once they return to the discussion, they ought to be able to behave more rationally.

Follow the rules of open and honest communication. In the initial stages of the confrontation there should be some ground rules established for effective communication. These rules constitute a verbal contract in which the participants make clear what they consider to be fair treatment. Whether each person will be able to "tell it like it is" and speak the truth regardless of the consequences will depend on mutual trust and the assurance that whatever is said will be kept confidential.

Basic rules to be followed in the name of fairness and courtesy are:

1. Each person should have opportunities to speak and express his/her thoughts. Others have the responsibility to listen carefully and respond in an appropriate manner.

2. The most effective response to another's comments is one given only after having listened to what was said, seeking input as needed for clarification, and then presenting your own thoughts on the statement.

Be alert to covert and manipulative behavior. The whole purpose of confrontation is to bring the problem out into the open; however, some people have trouble doing this. Consciously or unconsciously, they resort to undercover tactics to undermine their opposition. This kind of behavior has no place in a confrontation to resolve conflict.

Examples of manipulative and covert behavior are presented by deLodzia and Greenlaugh[22] as attempts to "get the other person." They include manipulation of *perceptions*, manipulation of *information*, and manipulation of *situations*.

Two techniques often used in the manipulation of perception are starting false rumors that put the other person in a bad light while the manipulator appears blameless; and sowing seeds of distrust in the minds of others so that they lose confidence in the opponent.

Manipulation of information can consist of withholding needed information from the opponent or hoarding it so that she appears foolish and incompetent. A third device that has the same effect is that of giving the opponent false information. Closely associated with these moves is the practice of "buttering up the boss," that is telling her what she wants to hear instead of honestly saying what she needs to hear.

Manipulation of situations is a far more complex "gaming" strategem in which all the above tactics and many more are used in an effort to alter the variables in the conflict situation.

These manipulative devices can be employed at any time, of course. They can be a cause of conflict as well as a result. When you suspect that such covert behavior is going on during attempts to resolve a conflict episode, you must intervene. Whether you choose dominance, persuasion, compromise, confrontation, or a combination of approaches to resolve the problem, you should have valid evidence that manipulative behavior is occurring.

In any case, do not allow yourself to be drawn into an interpersonal conflict and forced to take sides. If conflict between two persons is preventing honest dialogue and communication among group members, you may have to resolve that conflict before continuing with efforts to work with the group in confronting the original conflict episode.

It is very difficult to deal with several issues at once. All interpersonal conflict that carries over into the group will compound the issue under discussion and frustrate the goals of confrontation. In short, an interpersonal conflict involving two or more persons who are group members must be resolved before there can be a collaborative effort toward resolution of the larger conflict episode.

A confrontation with individual staff members who fail to meet required standards of performance is discussed in Chapter 10.

collaborative problem-solving

Confrontation is but the beginning of reaching conflict resolution through collaborative efforts. Once two or more individuals mutually identify a problem of conflict, they are ready to work together to plan for its resolution. Group problem solving has its advantages and its limitations, which were discussed in Chapter 5. The point to be emphasized here is that the resolution of a conflict episode *by the participants of the conflict* is more likely to have long-term and lasting results than if identification of the problem plans for resolution were developed by someone else and imposed on the conflict participants.

superordinate goals

Goals that are *mutually attractive* to each group in the conflict, and which *cannot be achieved* alone are called superordinate goals. Each group is dependent on the others for accomplishment of their goals.

Studies by Muzafer and Carolyn Sherif suggest that the increased contact and interdependence in the pursuit of superordinate goals facilitate reduction of intergroup conflict.[23] Nurse-managers who employ this technique to reduce conflict among various groups of employees under their supervision are likely to find that while conflict is not eliminated, it can be reduced to constructive levels and utilized to effect needed changes.

changing behavior patterns

Conventional methods for resolution of organizational conflict through education focus on the training of managers so that they can be more effective in accomplishing the goals of the organization. This approach does not take into consideration the altering of the hierarchical structure, its values, policies, and procedures. The basic assumption is that a change in interpersonal relations, especially those between managers and their subordinates, will result in a change in the organization and the resolution of conflict.

Traditional techniques for the development of management, as contrasted to organizational change, include programs of basic and continuing education that incorporate concepts of management, the behavioral sciences, and related disciplines. Educational programs are provided in a number of ways, either external to the organization or within it. Programs such as formal classes, seminars, and conferences conducted within and by the organization do not usually provide opportunities for the interaction of managers from a variety of settings outside the facility. The programs may be too much under the control of the administrators of the organization and therefore sheltered from the infusion of new ideas and fresh approaches to management's problems.

On the other hand, while programs outside the organization do allow for more interaction and exposure to innovative techniques of management, the participating managers may return from a stimulating learning experience eager and anxious to put into practice what they have learned, only to find that hierarchical structure, rules, and regulations prevent them from doing so.

Organization development (OD) researchers recommend several strategies to help deal with the problems encountered by managers who have learned newer, more humanistic management skills and techniques but are unable to implement them in an inflexible organizational structure. The most basic of these strategies is *sensitivity training* or *T-group training* in a laboratory setting away from familiar surroundings.

The goals of sensitivity training are many, but the essential ones are: (1) to develop self-awareness and sensitivity to others, (2) to assist participants in perceiving, and learning from the consequences of their behavior; (3) to assist them in understanding what their roles within the system are and how their roles are interrelated with other roles within the system; and (4) to help participants become more effective change agents.[24]

Evidence to support the effectiveness of sensitivity training as a means of improving interpersonal skills and reducing organizational conflict is still inconclusive. The major criticism against claims that such training will make organizations more adaptive to the needs of employees is that it alters only one of many interdependent variables in a highly complex system whose primary goal is cost-efficient production of either goods or services.

It is suggested that decentralization of authority and more whole-task division of work would effectively reduce conflict arising from the formal structure of the organization. If this is true, then nurse-managers must be skillful in delegating tasks, implementing change through group problem-solving, setting superordinate goals, and sharing decision making and conflict resolution with their subordinates. With this freedom to enjoy a higher level of autonomy comes shared responsibility and accountability on the part of every person on the nursing staff.

One of the major changes occurring in organized nursing services is, according to Brown, the decentralization of authority, fewer high-level administrators, and the transfer of more accountability for nursing care to the patient care units.[25]

HANDLING GRIEVANCES

In a conflict episode the complaints and grievances of employees are outward signs of the phase of manifest conflict. The employee perceives incompatibilities between his or her personal goals and needs and the policies and practices of the organization and its management.

Informal complaints and general griping are not the same as formal grievances, however. No job is so perfect that there are no complaints about minor irritations and dissatisfactions. Everyone at some time or other perceives the conflict in their employment situation. Personality clashes, generalized griping, and malcontent complaints are not considered to be legitimate grievances. If they become more specific and are directed toward what is perceived to be a breach of contract, then they become a legitimate grievance.

The term *grievance*, in the lexicon of labor relations experts, is a formal complaint made by an employee or group of employees under an established grievance procedure. The complaint may be made because of (1) an alleged violation of the application and interpretation of a clause in the contract between employee and employer; (2) managerial decisions that an employee or groups of employees consider to be arbitrary, capricious, and discriminatory; or (3) a management decision that violates precedents and past practices.[26]

Grievance procedures are advantageous to management because they provide a means of communication and often serve as a stimulus for the initiation and implementation of change.

Since 1974, when the Taft-Hartley Act was amended, personnel of nonprofit hospitals have the right to organize for purposes of collective bargaining through union representatives. Unionization and collective bargaining are seen by its advocates as the most effective means by which an employee or group of employees can present their point of view and draw attention to conditions that they perceive to be social injustices or disregard for their personal needs and goals. Formal grievance procedures are considered by union representatives to be one of the most important aspects of a labor union contract.

grievance procedures

Most institutions, unionized or not, have clearly defined grievance procedures. These are published in a policy manual or inhouse publication readily accessible to its employees. The procedure is a step-by-step guide, beginning with confrontation and informal discussions that usually are between the employee and his or her immediate supervisor, and ending with resolution or arbitration. The procedures give assurance to both labor and management that both sides of an issue are presented and efforts are made to resolve the conflict satisfactorily and productively.

First-line managers who are skillful in managing the conflict process often can avoid more formal grievance procedures. If they are skillful in the use of conflict strategems, disputes and discord among employees under their supervision can be mutually resolved without escalation into formal procedures involving higher levels of management. There may be times, however, when the settling of a grievance is beyond the power of a first-line manager. She must, after all, work within the structure of the organization and in conformity with existing policies and rules.

Grievances that are not settled informally are taken through the steps of the grievance procedure. The complainant may choose to go through the steps alone or with the help of a union or a professional organization representative. At each step an attempt is made to resolve the conflict. The final step of the process is arbitration and possibly negotiation of part or all of a new contract.

In institutions that are unionized, the negotiated contract between labor and management clearly describes the grievance procedure. It defines what a formal grievance is and outlines the manner in which it is to be presented to management. It also states the powers of an arbitrator and may describe the way in which the arbitrator is to be selected.[27]

guidelines for handling grievances

As a professional nurse and competent manager of patient care, you need not feel threatened by grievance procedures, even though the formal complaint may be against some action you have taken in your position of authority. As in any kind of confrontation, you need to behave assertively and positively. Communicate openly and honestly, and focus on the issue rather than personalities. Additionally, you should:

Approach the grievance procedure with the attitude that the problem will be resolved. It may, however, go all the way to arbitration involving representatives of both management and labor before a final settlement is reached.

Be prepared beforehand by becoming familiar with the contract, past practices and the kinds of decisions rendered in similar cases. Do not hesitate to ask for help from your supervisor.

Be prepared by documenting factual information that represents your position rationally and objectively. When preparing the data that you intend to present, check to be sure you have included each of the 5 W's. *Who* is the grievant? *What* is the specific nature of the grievance to be settled? *When* and *where* did the event or events related to the grievance take place? *Why* is the grievance being presented? This means what clause of the contract, managerial decision, past practice, precedent, policy, or rule does the grievant believe has been violated and what is your interpretation of the alleged violation. Finally, *how* do you think the situation can be rectified; what do you believe would be a fair and equitable solution?

Be persistent. Do not allow yourself to be sidetracked by irrelevant statements or intimidated by emotional attacks. Such measures might be tried, but you do not have to respond to them. Keep calm and cool, directing your statements to the issue being discussed and not to personal attacks. Don't allow yourself to become embroiled in a personality conflict.

Be flexible. Avoid painting yourself into a corner by being intransigent, insisting that your solution is the best and only one. An important aspect of negotiation and settlement is opportunity for each side to save face. A rigid and unyielding attitude during informal discussions greatly diminishes the possibility of reconciliation and face saving.

Keep in mind that there is always the chance that your decision will be reversed by management at a higher level. Do not take this personally, but resolve to learn from your mistakes and continue to work toward improving your problem-solving and decision-making skills. If, in the assessment of a problem, you find that resolution is beyond the scope of your authority, consult your supervisor.

REFERENCES

[1]Webster's Third International Dictionary, Encyclopedia Britannica, Inc., (Chicago: G. C. Merriam Co., 1971).

[2]K. Tye, "The Elementary School Principal: Key to Educational Change," in C. Culver, G. Hoban (eds.), *The Power to Change: Issues for the Innovative Education*, (New York: McGraw-Hill Book Co., 1973), p. 29.

[3]C. G. Smith, "A comparative analysis of some conditions and consequences of intraorganizational conflict," *Administrative Science Quarterly*, (March, 1966), p. 506.

[4]G. R. Pondy, "Organizational conflict: concepts and models," *Administrative Science Quarterly*, (Sept., 1967), pp. 296-320.

[5]J. H. Lewis, "Conflict management," *Journal of Nursing Administration*, (Dec., 1976), p. 53.

[6]W. Wohlking, "Organizational conflict and its resolution," *Supervisor Nurse*, (Oct., 1969), p. 17.

[7]B. Raven and A. Kruglanski, "Conflict and Power," in P. Swingle (ed.), *The Structure of Conflict*, (New York: Academic Press, 1970), pp. 70-72.

[8]M. Kramer and C. Schmalenberg, "Conflict: the cutting edge of growth," *Journal of Nursing Administration*, (Oct., 1976).

[9]H. R. Bobbitt, Jr., et al., *Organizational Behavior*, (Englewood Cliffs, N.J.: Prentice-Hall, Inc., 1974), p. 73.

[10]*A Review and Evaluation of Nursing Productivity*. R. C. Jelinek, Prin. Investigator and L. C. Dennis, Project Director, Health Manpower References, (U.S. Dept. of Health, Education, and Welfare. Bethesda, Md., Nov., 1976), p. 39.

[11]M. Leininger, "Conflict and conflict resolution," *Americal Journal of Nursing*, (Feb., 1975), p. 296.

[12]F. E. Kast and J. E. Rosenzweig, *Organization and Management*, (New York: McGraw-Hill Book Co., 1970), p. 294.

[13]R. Likert, *New Patterns of Management*, (New York: McGraw-Hill Book Co., 1961), p. 117.

[14]S. R. Robbins, *Managing Organizational Conflict*, (Englewood Cliffs, N.J.: Prentice-Hall, 1974), pp. 13-14.

[15]J. Lewis, *op cit.*, p. 54.

[16]G. deLodzia and L. Greenlaugh, "Recognizing change and conflict in a nursing environment," *Supervisor Nurse*, (June, 1973), p. 14.

[17]M. P. Follett, "Coordination," in Ed. H. F. Merrill *Classics in Management*, (New York: American Management Association, 1960), pp. 341-343.

[18]R. Veninga, "The management of conflict," *Journal of Nursing Administration*, (July-Aug., 1973), p. 32.

[19]R. Blake, H. Shepard and J. Mouton, *Managing Intergroup Conflict in Industry*, (Houston: Gulf Publishing Co., 1964), p. 67.

[20]G. O. Meyer, "Determinants of collective action attitudes among hospital nurses: an empirical test of a behavioral model," (University of Iowa, 1970).

[21]R. C. Myrtle and Eli Glogow, "How nursing administrators view conflict," *Nursing Research*, (March-April, 1978), pp. 103-106.

[22]G. deLodzia and L. Greenlaugh, *op cit.*, pp. 33-42.

[23]M. and C. Sherif, "Experiments in group conflict," *Scientific American*, (Nov., 1956), pp. 44-48.

[24]W. J. Duncan, *Essentials of Management*, (Hinsdale, Ill.: The Dryden Press, 1975), p. 449.

[25]E. G. Brown, *Nursing Reconsidered*, (Philadelphia: J. B. Lippincott Co., 1970), p. 68.

[26]E. Belerz and M. Meng, "The grievance process," *American Journal of Nursing*, (Feb., 1977), p. 256.

[27]*Ibid*, p. 259.

[28]The material in this section draws heavily from E. Berletz, *ibid.*, pp. 258, 259.

SUGGESTED READINGS

E. Beletz and M. Meng, "The grievance process," *American Journal of Nursing*, (Feb., 1977).

G. deLodzia and L. Greenlaugh, "Recognizing change and conflict in a nursing environment," *Supervisor Nurse*, (June, 1973).

M. Kramer and C. Schmalenberg, "Conflict: the cutting edge of growth," *Journal of Nursing Administration*, (Oct., 1976).

M. Leininger, "Conflict and conflict resolution," *American Journal of Nursing*, (Feb., 1975).

J. H. Lewis, "Conflict management," *Journal of Nursing Administration*, (Dec., 1976).

A. Marriner, "Conflict theory," *Supervisor Nurse*, (April, 1979).

A. Marriner, "Conflict resolution," *Supervisor Nurse*, (May, 1979).

R. C. Myrtle and E. Glogow, "How nursing administrators view conflict," *Nursing Research*, (March-April, 1978).

R. J. Plachy, "Head nurses: less griping, more action," *Journal of Nursing Administration*, (Jan., 1976).

P. K. Trinosky, "Nurse-doctor dissension still thrives," *Supervisor Nurse*, (April, 1979).

R. Veninga, "The management of conflict," *Journal of Nursing Administration*, (July-Aug., 1973).

W. Wohlking, "Organizational conflict and its resolution," *Supervisor Nurse*, (Oct., 1969).

chapter 10

index

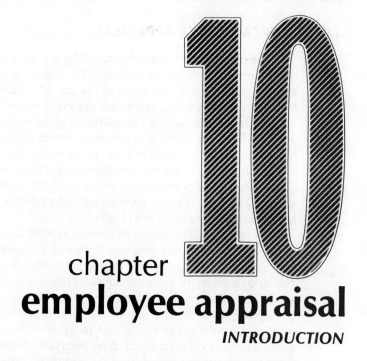

chapter

employee appraisal

INTRODUCTION

There was a time, in the not too distant past, when employee evaluations were conducted, recorded, and filed away in the personnel office without the employees ever having seen them. This was a fairly common practice in institutions where evaluations at least were done, albeit in a manner less than democratic. Some employees, especially technical and professional personnel, never have had an appraisal of their performance or suggestions for improvement.

In this chapter we will review the current trends in performance appraisal, recommended techniques for conducting formal evaluation programs, and approaches toward corrective and preventive action when there is evidence of unsatisfactory work. Emphasis has shifted from judgments about personal characteristics of an individual and subjective evaluations to measurable performance criteria and more objective tools for measuring whether or not the criteria are met.

Resistance to the whole notion of evaluating a subordinate's performance on the job has been due in large measure to the purposes for which they traditionally have been done and the lack of skill and confidence on the part of the person conducting the appraisal. It is hoped that a better understanding of purposes, techniques, and tools of measurement, coupled with a more democratic and humanistic approach, will make you more comfortable with the task of evaluating and improving the competence of your subordinates.

TRENDS IN EMPLOYEE APPRAISAL

The framework of components of the evaluation process are essentially the same regardless of the purposes for which the process is used or the kinds of information fed into the system. Consciously or unconsciously, formally or informally, judgments are made according to whether or not the subject of the evaluation measures up to expectations.

In a formal evaluation program or system of control, the basic components are: (1) the setting of criteria, goals, or expectations; (2) measurement of the subject of evaluation, whether it is performance or product or both; (3) comparison of performance or product with criteria; and (4) corrective action when there is a gap between desired performance and outcome, and actual performance or its end results.

Current trends in employee appraisal reflect a different way of looking at these four phases, the purposes for which they are used, and the manner in which appraisals are done. Traditionally, employee evaluation has been a system of control to meet the needs of the organization and its management. The employee being evaluated in the conventional mode is expected to accept passively the standards and expectations for performance developed by the organization and to agree with management's decisions about whether or not standards have been met. There are few opportunities for the employee to participate in the evaluation other than as the subject of the evaluation.

The newer approach refers to employee evaluation as a *systematic performance appraisal*. The implication is that it is not so much the person and his/her personal characteristics that should be measured as it is actual performance and the end results of that performance.

The newer terminology further implies that there is an orderly approach to the problem of evaluation and a capability for receiving and acting on feedback. The employee is actively engaged in all phases of the appraisal process. In essence, the new approach permits self-evaluation and encourages the development of independence and job maturity in the employee.

In Figure 10.1, adapted from a similar chart prepared by Dale Beach[1], differences between the conventional and newer approaches are summarized. As you can see, the two differ in terminology, purpose, target population, emphasis on the characteristic being evaluated, and the manner in which the appraisal interview between employee and manager is conducted.

In your particular employment situation you may be approaching the process in any of a number of ways. It is possible that employee evaluations are not being done at all, or at best are conducted in a haphazard, once-a-year, let's-get-it-over-with kind of way. Some of you might be engaged in a more organized and formalized program of periodic evaluation, but the approach is the conventional one that meets the needs of the organization and pays little attention to the personal needs and goals of each employee.

CONVENTIONAL MODE	SYSTEMATIC APPROACH
Terminology: Employee evaluation, efficiency report, fitness report, merit rating	*Terminology:* performance appraisal, employee appraisal
Purpose: Emphasis on wage increase, promotion, recommendation for employment elsewhere, and termination of employment	*Purpose:* Personal growth, increased competence, self-analysis and self-control
Designed for: Hourly paid workers	*Designed for:* Technicians and professionals
Characteristics emphasized: personal traits	*Characteristics emphasized:* outcome of performance, progress toward personal goals, measurement of behavior when performing tasks
Methodology: Rating by numbers, some room for comment. Comparison with workers performing a similar job	*Methodology:* Working with employee to set criteria for measuring performance and evaluating progress
Evaluation interview: Conducted at same time as discussion of job status, wages, etc. Evaluator's goal to have employee conform to organization's view of his job.	*Pre- and Post-appraisal interviews:* Conducted at time other than discussion of wages, promotion, etc. Evaluator encourages subordinate to set his own objectives in line with professional standards and criteria for performance

figure 10.1   trends in employee appraisal

The majority of staff nurses and their immediate supervisors view conventional employee evaluations as invalid, unreliable, and serving no useful purpose.[2] The criticisms may be well founded. Evaluations *are* a waste of time and damaging to the self-esteem of subordinates if they do not contribute to improvement of the quality of nursing care and the growth and development of the individuals who provide that care.

If you are among those who seriously and legitimately question whether employee evaluations are worthwhile, you might be interested in reviewing the purposes of evaluation from the perspectives of the subordinates being evaluated, their superiors, and administrators. The critical question is not whether you should waste your time taking part in an employee appraisal program. Observing your subordinates and evaluating both procedure and product or outcome in the delivery of nursing care is an appropriate and major task of the first-line supervisor. Your concern should be how to participate in a systematic appraisal program that contributes to more effective management of people and the development of their potential.

PURPOSES OF EMPLOYEE APPRAISAL

More than two decades ago Homer Kempfer wrote: "The basic purpose of evaluation is to stimulate growth and improvement . . . . Evaluation that does not lead to improved practice is sterile."[3]

Although he was writing about evaluation of education programs, Kempfer's words are equally relevant to employee appraisal programs. An intermediate goal or purpose of evaluation is to obtain information so that rational decisions can be made about current and future objectives and goals for the employee, management, and the total organization.

the subordinate's perspective

From the subordinate's point of view a properly conducted and effective appraisal program should:

- Guarantee fair and equitable treatment in regard to salary increases, promotions, and other kinds of recognition for achievement; and for reprimand, demotions and termination of employment when there is documented evidence of incompetence. An innate sense of fairness requires that people should be recognized for work well done. On the other hand, members of a work group resent the failure of management to do something about employees who are not doing their share of the work or who fail to meet standards of competence and conduct. If it makes no difference whether one performs well or poorly, morale suffers and motive forces are diminished.

- Provide a means by which subordinates can find out where they stand with respect to their job and in what particular areas of performance there is a need for change.

- Give opportunities for increased communication with the immediate supervisor for purposes of clarifying and integrating personal and organizational goals and objectives.

- Cause a subordinate to analyze his/her job and examine him/herself for strengths and weaknesses. Allow him/her to establish short term personal goals and accept responsibility for accomplishing them.[4]

In summary, an appraisal program does several things. It can provide an employee opportunities to satisfy needs and feel a sense of achievement, recognition and acceptance of responsibility. It can serve as a source of data to substantiate a request for advancement, and allow for more rational decision making when setting higher goals. You will recall that in his theory of motivation, Herzberg identified these factors as motivators or job satisfiers.[5] An employee who is able to participate in an appraisal program that is meaningful to him/her, is more likely to be motivated to improve and to find satisfaction in the work he/she is doing.

the manager's perspective

From your own perspective, formal and systematic performance appraisal can serve a number of useful purposes. First, it can motivate and guide you in the development of your own management skills. The current concepts of performance appraisal as we have been describing them were originally developed for application to management training and development. Helping someone else set personal goals and plan for their achievement is an excellent way to become more skillful in doing the same for yourself.

The data collected during systematic performance appraisal can be analyzed and organized so that it is useful to you for (1) identifying learning needs of your subordinates and validating requests for in-service education programs; (2) substantiate your recommendations for extrinsic and intrinsic rewards for competence or reprimand for incompetence; and (3) provide needed information for rational decision making in the delegation of tasks.

In Chapter 6 we discussed a leader's sources of power and influence. In his Position Power Rating Scale, Fiedler lists three questions related to evaluation and the leader's opportunity to directly or indirectly administer rewards and punishments and affect promotion, demotion, hiring, or firing of subordinates.[6] A negative answer to these questions indicates a weakness in the leader's power to influence subordinates. The implication is that if you do not actively participate in employee evaluations and do not wish to accept responsibility for making recommendations and providing rewards or reprimands according to the results of appraisals, you are denying yourself some of the power you need to function effectively as a manager.

the administrator's perspective

Organizations exist for the purpose of providing products and services more conveniently, reliably, and efficiently than independent agents can when functioning on their own. From the administrator's point of view, competent personnel are far more likely to achieve an organization's goals than are incompetent and unproductive workers. Controls and check points for determining efficiency and effectiveness are necessary to the operation of a smoothly running organizational system.

The systematic appraisal of employee performance is one part of an organization's system of control. Without any consideration for the humanistic aspects of management, it is good business sense to evaluate personnel, if for no other reason than to identify and reward productive workers and weed out the incompetent.

If, however, you add the more humanistic ingredient of concern for the development of each employee's potential for growth in his or her job, there is even more reason for a system of accountability and reward for achievement of goals. Supporters of a systematic appraisal program suggest that such a program is one way to accomplish the goals of administration by developing motivated and self-directed employees who are seeking personal goals of improvement integrated with organizational goals.

Nichols[7] did a study of 181 young nurses in military service and their perception of factors important to job satisfaction. She found that the nurses felt they would have been better satisfied with their job if they had (1) received information regarding evaluation of their work, (2) experienced impartial treatment of employees, and (3) received quality supervision. These items were perceived as important by more than 80 percent of the respondents, all of whom had worked as registered nurses for at least two years.

Job satisfaction and turnover of personnel are significantly related. People don't stay for very long in jobs that are intrinsically unrewarding, dissatisfying, and dead-ended. It is suggested that appraisal can be used to minimize the rate of avoidable turnover and maximize retention of competent nurses who would remain on the staff if they could accomplish some of their personal goals for growth in their jobs.[8,9] When properly planned and implemented, an appraisal program can meet professional and technical nurses' needs for recognition and achievement.

In terms of a cost-benefit analysis, it is less costly in time, effort, and money to implement an appraisal program that meets employees' needs than to recruit new staff nurses to fill vacancies. The waste of talent and expertise in nursing cannot be measured.

RESISTANCE TO EMPLOYEE APPRAISAL

There are two kinds of feelings that prevail in a first-line manager's resistance to employee evaluations: feelings of guilt and inadequacy. These feelings are the essence of the *felt conflict* phase described in Chapter 9. If you remember, the stage of felt conflict evolves from an awareness of conditions or factors in the environment that people become aware of and react to emotionally. Nurse-managers who resist evaluating their employees on a periodic and formal basis are reacting to an awareness of at least four factors relevant to the evaluation process: (1) complexity of the task, (2) lack of faith and trust in validity and reliability of the appraisal instrument, (3) discomfort in the role of judge, and (4) lack of self-confidence in handling appraisal interviews with employees.[10,11]

complexity of the task

In the evaluation of performance we are concerned with what the person does and the quality of the product, that is, the outcome of his/her performance of some aspect of work. It is difficult to measure these factors in an entity as vast and varied as nursing care. In recent years nurses have become increasingly more concerned about accountability and measurement of the outcome of the nursing process. Accountability implies the existence of standards and the measurement of both performance and outcome in terms of accepted standards.

In response to recognition of the need for a system of accountability the professional organizations in nursing have established and published standards to measure nursing care. Additionally, there are some extensively tested tools for measuring performance or outcome, or both. These reliable and valid tools are now in use in schools of nursing and in many different kinds of health care agencies and institutions. Three of the best known tools are: (1) *the Slater Nursing Competencies Rating Scale*, which measures the competencies of the individual nurse; (2) *the Quality Patient Care Scale (QualPacs)*, useful in an ongoing evaluation of the quality of patient care received in any setting in which there are nurse-patient interactions; and (3) *the Nursing Audit*, which is designed to measure the quality of care a patient has received during a specific cycle of care.

Although these tools are not completely objective, the persons making judgments about ratings are professional nurses. They observe the performance of a nurse while she is actively engaged in the nursing process, or they review patients' charts for documentation of the care provided by nurses and the evidence of that care.[12]

The major characteristics of these and similar valid and reliable tools for evaluation are that they require either direct observation of the persons being evaluated or a review of the data that provide evidence of the results of performance. Items on these instruments indicate *specific behaviors that are measurable to some degree*.

When you are preparing to engage in the evaluation of an employee you must make some decisions about the specific areas of competence that you intend to measure in a given time. In other words, you must decide exactly *what will be measured, when*.

Ideally, these decisions are made with each employee, taking into consideration his/her specific needs for improvement. Even if you must work with a printed form that is general in its list of items to be measured, you can narrow down the area in which you and your employee think there is need for improvement. Concentrate on changing specific behaviors in regard to learning new skills or upgrading performance so that it is more in line with expectations listed in the employee's job description and more compatible with the objectives of your particular patient care unit.

Job descriptions have come in for their share of criticism from behaviorists who see it as too confining, useless in making plans for improvement, and stifling of creativity and enthusiasm for the job. While there is some truth in this, the fact remains that personal goals must be integrated with goals of the patient care unit and the organization. Individuality can be tolerated up to a point, but the vast majority of work is best accomplished in an orderly and structured environment. Job descriptions that are prepared according to the concepts of management by objectives (MBO) and appraisal by results (APR) can be very helpful in determining criteria for employee appraisal.[13] Admittedly, a performance description is not a perfect tool for employee evaluation, but it can provide a sound basis for the development of realistic and practical standards of performance for different levels of nursing.

The more clearly you can define expectations, the more easily you can determine whether expectations are being met. The complex task of appraisal in nursing cannot be done as a whole and all at one time. It is in the accumulating of small truths that we arrive at a larger truth. Appraisal must be broken into small increments that represent realistic and measurable steps in an employee's progress toward the overall goal of improved practice.

lack of faith and trust in the instrument

In the terminology of evaluators, an *instrument* is the set of factors or characteristics being measured and the means by which they are given a rating or grade. A written test given in a course of study is an instrument for measuring progress in learning the content of that course. In the traditional approach to appraisal of employees, an instrument for measurement usually is some kind of printed form prepared by the personnel department. Quality and quantity of work, knowledge of job, dependability, and attendance, are some of the items commonly found on a conventional employee rating instrument. The evaluator uses these forms to give the employee a numerical rating on a scale of 1 to 5 or 1 to 10.

validity

The *validity* of an instrument is an indication of the extent to which it does the job for which it is used. If an employee appraisal instrument or tool leads to improved practice of nursing because it leads to a higher level of competence in the person whose performance has been evaluated, it can be said to be a valid instrument. The validity of an instrument is specific to the purposes for which it is used. Thus, the term can have different meanings, depending on why and how it is used for evaluation.

The evidence used to verify the validity of an instrument must be appropriate to the stated purpose. A manager may use an evaluation form to substantiate her claims that a particular employee is incompetent. The evidence that she presents on the form must point to incompetence in specific areas of practice and not to personality or some other personal characteristic that the manager finds displeasing. If the instrument does not measure competence in the performance of one's job, it cannot be said to be a valid tool for performance appraisal.

Unfortunately, many of the instruments used in the conventional approach to employee evaluations are not valid from the subordinate's point of view. They do not lead to improved practice; do not tell the employee specifically where there is need for improvement in job performance; do not provide for increased communication between the subordinate and his/her immediate supervisor, or allow for the setting of short term personal goals and acceptance of responsibility for accomplishing them.

From the manager's point of view, they do not help identify specific learning needs of employees, nor are they noted for their usefulness in providing motivation and job satisfaction. In fact, many evaluation programs that require the exclusive use of conventional instruments have the opposite effect precisely because they do not serve the same purposes as a systematic and process-oriented, participative appraisal. Problems arise because an out-dated tool is being used to try to do a job that can be done much better by an instrument that is specially designed to accomplish more up-to-date goals and purposes.

reliability

The *reliability* of an instrument has to do with the extent to which it is *consistent* in measuring whatever it purports to measure. A reliable instrument is dependable and stable. It gives similar results in the hands of a number of different people and continues to do so over a period of time and with a variety of subjects being tested.

The criteria of a reliable instrument are not subject to a variety of interpretations by the persons using the instrument. This reduces the possibility of human error on the part of the rater. For example, an instrument that reliably measures knowledge and skill in the emergency care of a patient in acute respiratory distress would give the same rating to all persons who were competent in this area of practice. The rating for the performance of a particular person would be the same when used by several different professional evaluators observing and rating that person's competence.

The distrust and lack of faith in the validity and reliability of the instruments traditionally used to measure competence in nursing has come about as a result of many nurses' experience with them as students and as staff nurses. They realize that it is rather ridiculous to give a numerical rating to such affective factors as cooperation, initiative, attitude, and interest. They also are aware that the numerical ratings do not in truth provide help for setting goals for improvement, nor do they have much meaning to anyone who has not observed specific behaviors of the person who received the ratings.

There should be no reason why you must confine your appraisal activities to completing evaluation forms that you have no faith in and do not trust to be valid and reliable. You can engage your subordinates in an appraisal program that is geared toward their needs for improvement and more able to serve the purposes for which an appraisal program should be conducted. The beauty of such a program is that it encourages each staff member to be in competition with herself, rather than with others who are working at the same or a different level of practice.

discomfort in the role of judge

First-line managers in nursing usually are not very comfortable about judging the behavior of others. They are fully aware of the relationship among competent nurses and the quality of nursing care received by patients, but they also are sensitive to human needs for self-esteem, security, and acceptance by others. An approach to employee evaluation that emphasizes personal characteristics that are poorly defined and subject to interpretation and human error is an affront to their sense of fairness and respect for human dignity and the personal worth of every individual.

McGregor views the reluctance of managers to participate in employee appraisal programs as a "deep but unrecognized wisdom" that tells them it just doesn't seem right to make judgments on the basis of insufficient and invalid evidence. He points out that most appraisal plans not only require managers to make these judgments but also to sit down and tell their subordinates how they have been judged.[14]

It is suggested that the resolution of this interpersonal conflict can be found in the newer and more humanistic approach previously defined and summarized in Table 10.1. This approach takes you out of the role of judge and places you in the position of guide and facilitator.

lack of confidence in handling appraisal interviews

Many managers feel unsure of themselves during appraisal interviews because they realize how important evaluations can be to employees. They hesitate to say or do anything that could be damaging to the individual's sense of dignity and personal worth. When evaluations are conducted only once or twice a year, are focused mainly on personality traits, and are written mostly as subjective numerical ratings, it is not easy to defend the ratings that are given. A more humanistic approach can reduce some of the anxiety about discussing appraisals with employees. However, whatever approach is made to the problem of appraisal, some judgments must be made at the time actual performance is compared with standards or critical expectations for performance.

Decisions about the quality of work performed by a subordinate are subject to personal bias and other human errors and organizational influences. If you can avoid some of these errors and influences you will be less uncomfortable in your role as guide and counselor and be better able to give your subordinates an honest opinion about how they are meeting standards and where they could improve.

The errors that raters most often commit are human errors to which we are all susceptible. Appraisal is a human endeavor and some personal feelings and memories of past experiences are bound to influence our perception of the behavior of others. If we were measuring inanimate objects with perfectly reliable and valid tools, there would be no problem with errors of subjectivity. But people are not objects, and evaluation of human behavior is difficult at best. The more common errors and problems likely to develop during the appraisal process are summarized in Figure 10.2. You will be more confident and more comfortable when you conduct appraisal interviews if you have tried your best to avoid these errors.

Another factor that could contribute to feelings of inadequacy is the problem of discussing salary increases, taking corrective disciplinary action in cases of incompetence, and other activities related to the conferring of rewards and reprimands on the basis of evaluations. It is strongly recommended by advocates of the newer approach to employee appraisals that these subjects not be discussed at the same time that you are talking with a subordinate about his/her personal goals. Disciplinary interviews should not be confused with an appraisal or developmental interview. The two are conducted for different purposes and require different kinds of interpersonal skills and attitudes.

It is inevitable that not all members of your staff will be able to function at the desired level. When this happens, you should be able to recommend some kind of action that will prevent the incompetent person from jeopardizing the welfare of your patients. But this kind of problem will be discussed later when we talk about corrective action. For the present, we are concerned with improving your skill and confidence in using a goal-oriented approach to employee appraisal.

ERROR	WHAT HAPPENS?	WHEN IS IT LIKELY TO OCCUR?
Personal Bias	Rater allows the way he/she feels about a person to influence the rating of performance.	When objective measurement is difficult, as in interpersonal skills, attitude, etc.; or, when the tool being used does not contain measurable and behavior-centered criteria.
Organizational influences	Rater makes appraisal according to the use that will be made of the results. If used for wage increase, recommendations for future jobs, etc., the employee receives a high rating. If used for improvement of the person's competence, the rating is lower and weaknesses are emphasized.	When rater is overly concerned about the ego needs of the subordinate. This is considered to be a natural inclination, but it does suggest subjectivity.
Central tendency	Rater gives everyone an average or middle score.	When rater does not have sufficient data to make a judgment about performance, or when results of the appraisal are to be used for organizational purposes.
Leniency	Rater gives everyone a high rating.	When the tool being used does not require objective data and rater is unsure of her ability to evaluate employees. Commonly occurs when only one person does the rating.
Strictness	Rater gives everyone a low rating.	Organization influences demand that employees not receive high ratings. Personal feelings about individual being rated.
Halo effect	Rater scored every trait high or low because of personal like or dislike. Rating of one characteristic influences rating of other characteristics.	Subjective interpretations of the rater. Error of logic. If employee is competent in one area, she must be competent in others.

figure 10.2   common errors and problems in rating

IMPLEMENTING AN APPRAISAL PROGRAM

Although systematic appraisal programs based on individual needs and goals of the employee have long been advocated by management specialists, they are not being used yet in many health care agencies and organizations. Without going into the reasons why this is so, we can be encouraged by the enthusiasm with which many nurse-managers greet the news that there is an alternative to the traditional methods of evaluation with which they are so uncomfortable. Regardless of the kind of program in effect in the organization in which you work, you should be able to work with each of your subordinates to develop a plan that will help meet his/her needs and short-term career goals.

If you think about it for a moment, you will see that there are certain similarities between developing a nursing care plan for a patient and developing an individualized employee appraisal plan. Both are participative endeavors requiring active involvement of the person for whom the plan is being developed. The appraisal process is continuous and responsive to the needs that are identified throughout the process.

As you well know, the development of a plan to meet individual needs requires a high level of knowledge and skills and an attitude of commitment. Planning takes time, patience, and perseverance. Implementing the plan and evaluating its effectiveness demands the same commitment. Throughout the process internal and external environmental conditions will change and human errors and foibles will create a certain amount of frustration and conflict.

Many nurses are still resisting the development of nursing care plans for their patients in spite of an abundance of credible evidence to support the belief that such plans are beneficial to the nurses and their patients. Stevens[15] suggests that this resistance arises from conceptual and operational problems. Many nurses have been taught that a correct decision leads to *the* correct outcome. They are under the impression that the scientific method of decision making, when applied to problems, will produce predictable outcomes in every instance. The variable of human interaction in nursing and in the management of people greatly reduces the certainty that what is planned will be achieved. This uncertainty need not interfere with your commitment to the development of an appraisal plan for your employees. You simply need to be aware of the element of risk in putting something on paper, then having to revise it because of extenuating circumstances.

Once you are committed, at least in principle, to the concept of individualized employee appraisals, your next concern should be the practical or operational aspects of the task. What special skills do you need? What specific knowledge should you have in order to function in the role of guide, facilitator, and counselor? There is no doubt that the task is complex, but you already are familiar with the concept of process and the phases of assessment, planning, implementation, and evaluation.

PREPARATION FOR EMPLOYEE APPRAISAL

In their study of thousands of people in varying levels of management, Laughlin and Kedzie found that employees want guidance in how to do better the things they don't do well. They want specific suggestions for improvement rather than generalities about unsatisfactory performance. And, they prefer that the appraisal be a continuous process in which they can participate under the direction of and in communication with a knowledgeable supervisor.[16]

Because of your position in the organization, it is your responsibility to assume the role of leader and to maintain an appropriate level of authority and control throughout the appraisal process. Allowing an employee to set personal goals and working with him/her to achieve them does not mean abrogating your position as leader. Being overly concerned about democratic principles and participative management can be a disservice to your subordinates, yourself, and your patients.

standards and criteria

Employees expect a knowledgeable supervisor to be a source of information about the standards and criteria against which their performance will be measured. Some resources for this kind of information that should be readily available in your office files are listed below.

- Copies of job descriptions for each level of the nursing staff on your unit.

- Copies of the printed evaluation forms or tools of measurement required by the personnel department and the department of nursing. These forms should reflect differences in the various levels of nursing. You do not use the same criteria to evaluate the performance of nurse attendants, practical nurses, and registered nurses; therefore, you should have a different appraisal instrument for each of these groups.[17] If the organization provides only one form for all levels of nursing, you should devise some way by which you can differentiate expectations validly and reliably.

- Copies of the goals and objectives of the nursing department and the specific nursing care objectives of your patient care unit. An MBO (management by objectives) approach is easily integrated into the appraisal process.[18]

- A copy of the American Nurses Association standards of nursing care, especially those that are specific to the population of patients cared for in your unit. It also could be helpful to have other published standards and criteria such as those published by the National League for Nursing and the Joint Commission for Accreditation of Hospitals. If you are working in an agency of distributive nursing rather than episodic care there are some governmental agencies and public health departments that publish standards for health care in clinics and neighborhood health care centers.

- A copy of the Nursing Practice Standards for Licensed Practical/ Vocational Nurses, adopted by the National Federation of Licensed Practical Nurses House of Delegates in Oct., 1979; and a copy of the Code of Ethical Practice and Conduct for Licensed Practical/ Vocational Nurses adopted by the NFLPN in 1961 and revised in 1979.

- A copy of the Working Paper of the NLN Task Force on Competencies of Graduates of Nursing Programs (NLN Pub. No 14-1787), available from the Publications Order Unit, NLN, 10 Columbus Circle, New York, N.Y., 10019. Payment of $1.50 each must accompany orders of $10 or less.

  The publication represents efforts to define and distinguish the competencies or minimal expectations of new graduates from the four types of nursing programs. It is a series of models that compare and contrast the knowledge base and practice role of the four types of nursing graduates.

accountability and reward system

Two essential elements of an effective performance appraisal program are an accountability system and a reward system.[19] Accountability means merely that one is held responsible for his/her performance and its consequences. A properly designed appraisal program recognizes both achievement and failure to meet standards of performance. A reward system provides some means by which an employee is rewarded intrinsically and extrinsically for accomplishing personal and organizational objectives and goals.

It may be that your organization or agency has a merit raise system whereby employees automatically receive monetary benefits when their work is rated above average or higher than critical expectations. When such a system is in effect, you should be sure that your subordinates know about and fully understand how merit increases are earned. Other kinds of extrinsic rewards include promotions, increase in status, and a higher level of autonomy.

Even though you may not be able to directly influence the dispensing of extrinsic rewards, you ought to be able to make recommendations for recognition of achievement. Additionally, you can provide intrinsic rewards for performance that is satisfactory. Frequent comments about a subordinate's progress can be an effective form of positive reinforcement, as can statements about the importance of his/her contribution to overall team effort and the accomplishment of the objectives of the patient care unit. Special awards presented in a way that publicly recognizes exceptional performance should be reserved for outstanding work; otherwise they lose their motivational effectiveness.

You can help each employee to prepare for the appraisal process by helping him/her become familiar with the functional job description and the standards by which the quality of nursing care is evaluated on your patient care unit. Several authorities recommend that the first order of business in an employee appraisal is informing each subordinate what is expected. Some suggest that the appraisal process starts the first day of employment during orientation.[20] Although some general orientation usually is done by the department of staff development or in-service education, this does not take the place of a personal orientation to the patient unit. The employee's immediate supervisor is responsible for discussing job descriptions, evaluation forms, performance standards, unit objectives, and other job expectations with each subordinate.

Once orientation to the unit is completed, you should ask the employee to prepare specific short term goals based on his/her self-assessment and the identification of specific needs for growth in the job, and improvement of professional expertise.[21] These specific and personal goals should be written down and brought to the planning session at the beginning of the appraisal process.

The introduction of a new appraisal system for employees who have been working with you over a period of time will require slightly different strategems. You cannot assume that those who have been evaluated under an old system already know about job expectations and are fully prepared to start setting their own goals for improvement.

AN EXAMPLE OF PERFORMANCE APPRAISAL

Ms. May has been head nurse of a 43-bed medical unit in a 300-bed acute-care facility for three years. During the past year she has been using a new employee appraisal system introduced by the nursing department and in effect in every patient care unit in the organization. Ms. May was comfortable with the system because it emphasized performance and the setting of personal goals for her subordinates. She has developed a complete file of the resources needed to familiarize each employee with his/her job description, acceptable standards of care and critical expectations for job performance.

When Tim White, a recent graduate with a BSN was hired to work on Ms. May's unit, he was oriented by in-service education staff members for a full week. During that time he completed a self-assessment form on which he identified nursing procedures that he felt confident in performing and those he was less sure about. He was not as confident of his ability to perform in the implementation phase of the nursing process as in the assessment and planning phases.

During their first session together, Ms. May talked with Tim about his self-assessment, his past experiences in nursing and his interests outside nursing. She reviewed Tim's job description with him and went over the objectives for the patient care unit. He was asked to prepare a list of personal goals that he would like to accomplish in the next six weeks.

The second session took place after Tim had been introduced to the staff members he would be working with, and had become familiar with the kinds of patients admitted to the unit, the most frequent nursing procedures performed, equipment used, and the location of supplies, and so forth. He discussed with Ms. May the list of goals that he had prepared. He wanted to improve his competence in such procedures as passing nasogastric tubes, suctioning tracheostomies, starting intravenous fluids, and administering medications. He also wanted to develop skill in dealing with nurse attendants and practical nurses, especially in regard to delegating tasks and follow-up.

Ms. May accepted Tim's goals for improvement and together they planned for their achievement. She agreed to:

- Find opportunities for Tim to perform the nursing procedures he had listed and arrange for him to be observed by herself or an experienced RN on the staff. They would use a checklist during observation and rate his performance as satisfactory or unsatisfactory.

- Conduct an ongoing performance appraisal to determine other needs he might not be aware of. Specific areas of performance would include nursing procedures, charting and attention to patient needs. In regard to Tim's leadership skills, she agreed to observe his performance in making assignments and eliciting cooperation from those who worked under his direction.

- Gather data by such techniques as anecdotal records, checklists, input from peers and co-workers, and documented evidence of patient response to the care he provided.

Tim's part in the agreement was that he would: (1) review the procedures in the nursing manual and prepare himself for performing them; (2) willingly perform a procedure when told that there was an opportunity to do so; (3) evaluate his own performance; (4) read at least one article on delegation and one on modular nursing recommended by the in-service education department; (5) help gather data about his performance so that a meaningful appraisal could be done at the end of the six weeks.

During the period of appraisal Ms. May met with Tim to inform him of her findings and allow him to express his thoughts about his progress. The meetings were brief and arranged at times when either party felt a need to discuss the appraisal.

At the end of the six weeks an appraisal interview was held with Tim. He had made satisfactory progress toward achievement of most of his goals. He found that he needed to improve his nursing care plans because there was evidence that they were too elaborate and not always followed by the other nurses. He was not comfortable in a leadership role in his dealings with nurse attendants and practical nurses, and he agreed that his documentation of patient care and patient education needed improvement. New goals were set and plans made for their achievement within three months.

Tim's progress was satisfactory and he was able to assess his needs for improvement under the direction of the head nurse. Not every subordinate will be able to do this and some may show no progress. When there is evidence of incompetence and no signs of improvement over a reasonable period of time, corrective action may be necessary.

CORRECTIVE ACTION

The fourth phase of the appraisal process is corrective action to eliminate any discrepancy between expectations and reality. The corrective action can be focused on the performance and its outcome or it can involve a revision of the criteria or standards. Sometimes during evaluation it becomes apparent that the expectations stated at the beginning of the process prove to be unattainable, too difficult to measure, or unrealistic because of conditions beyond the control of the individuals involved.

At the other extreme there may be standards of performance that are so low they do not present a challenge. You will remember that in Chapter 9 it was pointed out that there should be some degree of conflict to provide impetus for a change for the better. Employees who are not challenged to improve are not much better off than those who are frustrated by unrealistic goals that cannot possibly be achieved.

In general, criteria that apply to groups of employees working at a certain level should not be changed unless there is sufficient reason to do so. Some expectations of performance, such as those stated in personnel policies, professional nursing organization standards, and organizational goals, are not subject to major change by a first-line supervisor. Individualized criteria that represent personal goals of an employee will change as the employee shows progress and growth in his/her practice of nursing.

critical and desirable outcomes

When criteria for employee performance are developed for the varying levels of nursing staff members, it is necessary to differentiate between *critical expectations* and those that are more *desirable*. Critical expectations represent the minimum or satisfactory level of performance.[22] For example, the use of sterile technique in the performance of certain nursing procedures is a must; it is a critical expectation that cannot be changed or compromised. All patients have the right to be safe from contamination through carelessness or ignorance. All registered and licensed practical nurses are expected to know about and observe principles of sterile technique. The expectation that nurses will not compromise principles of medical and surgical asepsis is a critical, rather than a desirable criterion. The expectation that they will insist on cleanliness and handwashing on the part of nurse attendants and other nonprofessional personnel is highly desirable.

Members of the nursing staff of an organization are expected to follow its policies regarding tardiness and absence from work. Some allowances will be made in the policy for occasional and unavoidable lateness and absence, but these represent minimum standards that cannot be changed to suit the needs and goals of individuals. It is desirable that every employee report to work on time each day and have no absences, but the expectation for a perfect record is desirable rather than critical.

Whenever criteria that apply to a group of employees are changed, as in changes in procedure and policy, everyone affected should be notified so that they fully understand the new criteria by which they will be evaluated.

correcting performance deficiencies

Corrective action resulting from failure to meet performance standards and criteria usually is thought of in terms of firing, reprimand, suspension, and other kinds of punitive action. Though there will be occasions when these measures are necessary to protect patients, preserve morale, and maintain order in the working environment, there are other approaches that are less harsh and oftentimes more effective.

Research studies have shown that not knowing how to perform as expected is one of the major reasons for disciplinary action. Punishing people for a lack of information or undeveloped skills is the least desirable way to get them to improve. Insufficient knowledge and skill in the performance of some nursing tasks could be the result of lack of experience in a particular area of clinical nursing practice. With proper instruction and supervised practice a staff member should be able to make up specific deficiencies relatively quickly and easily.

There is a limit, however, to the amount of time and effort you can expend trying to help an employee meet critical expectations. It is not unreasonable to expect credentialed nursing personnel to be able to function effectively at a particular level. Registered nurses, licensed practical nurses, and trained nurse attendants have all received some kind of formal teaching in preparation for employment. Each level of nursing has its lower and upper limits and some overlapping of tasks. When an employee's performance goes well beyond the limits established by the job description, you have no choice but to take some corrective action other than continued efforts to instruct and guide the employee.

disciplinary action

A decision to take some disciplinary action should not happen on the spur of the moment when you are exasperated and emotionally distraught with an employee's failure to do her share of the work and to do it competently. If you postpone dealing with the problem until it becomes critical, you are more likely to react to some relatively minor incident and launch into a tirade for which you will later feel guilty. Instead of overreacting emotionally you want to deal with the problem rationally and assertively.[23]

If you are hesitant to take some disciplinary action even though it is plainly called for, you are not alone in that feeling. Disciplinary action is not popular among managers. In his study of employee relations, Wohlking cites several reasons why managers do not discipline their subordinates. Among these reasons are: (1) they don't know how to handle discipline problems and conduct disciplinary interviews; (2) they rationalize their behavior by saying to themselves, why tell an employee what he/she has done wrong when he/she already knows what should have been done or not done, or, why should I discipline employees when no one else does; and (3) they may not believe that higher levels of management will back up a disciplinary action.[24]

Rationalizations are not valid excuses for doing what you know should be done. The belief that employees already know how they have failed to meet expectations may or may not be based on facts. If employees have not been participants throughout the process, they may not know what they have done wrong or where they have failed to do what they should. Corrective action should be taken only after an employee has been fully informed of expectations, had his/her performance evaluated, and had opportunities to discuss any discrepancies between performance and expectations. If there is a question about whether or not an employee really knows where he/she has failed, the best thing to do is sit down with him/her and confront the problem.

The excuse that no one else disciplines employees, whether true or not, is completely beside the point. What other people do or don't do should not influence your decision to behave as an effective manager. The reluctance of someone else to discipline employees does not relieve you of your responsibility to take actions that you know to be in the best interest of your patients.

In regard to the handling of discipline problems and support and backing from higher levels of management, you will need to be skillful in dealing with conflict and maintaining good communications with your superiors. A discipline problem should be analyzed to determine its nature and precisely what it is that you are dealing with.[25] How serious is the problem? Are critical expectations not being met or is it a matter of wanting the employee to perform exceedingly well and meet highly desirable criteria? How long has the employee failed to perform as expected? Is a pattern developing, or are there isolated incidents that could be due to circumstances beyond the employee's control, as for example, understaffing, emergencies, and so on? How much help has been given to the employee to improve competence and meet criteria of performance?

Organizations usually have some policies and procedures to be followed when disciplinary action is necessary. You will need to know about these and to discuss your specific problem with your supervisor. You ought to be confident that whatever action you decide to take, there will be a good chance that your decision will not be reversed by administration should the employee decide to make an appeal.

After you have identified the problem and decided that some action should be taken to correct the situation, you will need to decide what that action will be. Fleishman suggests that there are four principles applicable to corrective action in the appraisal process.[26] Disciplinary action should be:

1. Equitable, that is, appropriate to the nature of the problem as identified through analysis.

2. Prompt and firm, gradually progressing from less severe to more severe measures. Most authors recommend that the progression should be from oral warning, to written warning, to suspension, to dismissal or termination of employment. Your organization may already have a policy regarding the steps to be taken and how disciplinary actions should be documented.

3. Based on factual evidence of unacceptable behavior.

4. Applied consistently without bias or favoritism.

After you have decided on the kind of disciplinary measure that you will take to deal with the problem, and discussed the problem and your decision with your immediate supervisor, your next step is to conduct a disciplinary interview with the employee. In effect, the interview is a confrontation with the issue of incompetence and a conflict between personal goals and organizational goals. During the interview you will need to keep the discussion focused on the issue and not allow peripheral topics such as personal problems, to be brought into the dialogue with the employee.

It is at this point that nurses often lose sight of the goals and purposes of the interview. You should not confuse working relationships with your employees and therapeutic relationships with your patients or clients.[27] Personal problems outside the working environment that are interfering with an employee's performance are regrettable, but a subordinate should not expect you to accept these problems as a valid excuse for failure to meet the standards and goals of the organization and the objectives of your patient care unit. You may be able to refer an employee to a professional person or agency who can help resolve his/her problems, but in your role as manager the employee is your subordinate and not your client. If you abrogate your responsibilities as manager and become involved in problems over which you have no control, the ultimate outcome may very well be that it is your patients who suffer the consequences.

With experience you will become more comfortable with disciplinary interviews. Corrective action does not always entail some kind of reprimand. In fact, if the process is carried out as a cooperative effort with improvement as its goal, warnings, suspension, and dismissal should not be necessary except on rare occasions when employees are not able to improve or are not motivated to do so.

REFERENCES

[1]D. S. Beach, *Personnel—The Management of People at Work*, 2nd ed, (New York: The MacMillan Co. 1970), p. 310.

[2]"Job evaluations: giving and getting them with less of a hassle," *Nursing '75*, (Nov., 1975), pp. 75-80.

[3]H. Kempfer, *Adult Education*, (New York: McGraw-Hill, 1955), p. 399.

[4]D. McGregor, "An uneasy look at performance appraisal," *Harvard Business Review*, (Sept.-Oct., 1972).

[5]F. Herzberg, *The Motivation to Work*, (New York: Wiley & Sons, Inc., 1959).

[6]F. Fiedler, et al., *Improving Leadership Effectiveness*, (New York: John Wiley and Sons, Inc., 1976), p. 149.

[7]G. A. Nichols, "Important, satisfying, and dissatisfying aspects of nurses' jobs," *Supervisor Nurse*, (Jan., 1974), pp. 10-15.

[8]T. R. Tirney and N. Wright, "Minimizing the turnover problem," *Supervisor Nurse*, (Aug., 1973), pp. 47-58.

[9]R. D. Gauerke, "Appraisal as a retention tool," *Supervisor Nurse*, (June, 1973), pp. 37-42.

[10]I. G. Ramey, "Setting standards and evaluating care," *Journal of Nursing Administration*, (May-June, 1973).

[11]D. McGregor, *op. cit.*

[12]M. A. Wandelt, et al., "Tools for evaluation," *Hospital Topics*, (Aug., 1972).

[13]C. Gerald, "Is the position description obsolete?," *Hospital Progress*, (May, 1971).

[14]D. McGregor, *op. cit.*

[15]B. J. Stevens, "Why won't nurses write nursing care plans?," *Journal of Nursing Administration*, (Nov./Dec., 1972).

[16]T. C. Laughlin and D. P. Kedzie, "What employees want in an appraisal," *Best's Review*, (July, 1971), p. 37.

[17]D. del Bueno, "Implementing a performance evaluation system," *Supervisor Nurse*, (Feb., 1979), p. 43.

[18]C. Golightly, "MBO and performance appraisal," *Journal of Nursing Administration*, (Sept., 1979), p. 11.

[19]D. del Bueno, *op cit.*

[20]H. Mayfield, "In defense of performance appraisal," *Harvard Business Review*, (March-April, 1960).

[21]N. West, M. Ayers, and J. Sudbury, "An objective appraisal instrument for nurses," *Supervisor Nurse*, (March, 1979), p. 32.

[22]D. del Bueno, *op. cit.*

[23]M. Chenevert, *Special Techniques for Assertiveness Training*, (St. Louis: C. V. Mosby Co., 1978), p. 72.

[24]W. Wohlking, "Effective discipline in employee relations," *Personnel Journal*, (Sept., 1975).

[25]*Ibid.*

[26]R. Fleishman, "Disciplinary action: friend or foe?," *Supervisor Nurse*, (June, 1978), p. 30.

[27]M. Chenevert, *op. cit.*, p. 74.

SUGGESTED READINGS

A. P. Brief, "Developing a usable performance appraisal system," *Journal of Nursing Administration*, (Oct., 1979).

G. F. Dau, "The appraisal process," *Supervisor Nurse*, (Aug., 1976).

D. del Bueno, "Implementing a performance appraisal system," *Supervisor Nurse*, (Feb., 1979).

J. Engle, "The evaluation of a public health nursing performance evaluation tool," *Journal of Nursing Administration*, (April, 1979).

A. Finkelman, "The standards of nursing practice and the supervisor," *Supervisor Nurse*, (May, 1976).

R. Fleishman, "Disciplinary action: friend or foe?," *Supervisor Nurse*, (June, 1978).

C. Golightly, "MBO and performance appraisal," *Journal of Nursing Administration*, (Sept., 1979).

B. Lawson, "Evaluation—a sorry procedure," *Supervisor Nurse*, (Sept., 1978).

A. Marriner, "Evaluation of personnel," *Supervisor Nurse*, (May, 1965).

index

Folios in italics refer to Suggested Readings